I0789612

Love Trust Gratitude Healing

Turning a Battle into a Dance and making Peace with Cancer

Cover Design by Alexander von Ness

There is little justice in the world, yes, life isn't fair. The counterbalance to an unfair unjust world lies within us and is manifested by the quality of our response when unfairness or injustice comes our way.

****

In life there are events that strike us with such force they alter reality itself and come to be recognized as a before and after. The sudden passing of a beloved, a car accident that leaves one paralyzed are a couple examples. A cancer diagnosis is another.

On the morning of April 12, 2018, I got out of bed expecting as always to stand and walk across the room. Instead my legs gave way and I crumpled to the floor. My reaction was curious disbelief. As I was going down I thought, Huh, what is this? This can't be. The impact of my fall woke my wife Jen who asked, "What happened?" "I fell," I answered, as I struggled to my hands and knees, shaky and weak, yet certain I could shift my right foot under me and stand up. I couldn't. Jen sat up in bed and turned on the light next to her. "Are you okay?" "I don't know." I dropped my head and stared at my legs trying to will them into action. It was beyond belief that they wouldn't obey my simple command. I noticed numbness growing in my legs. It was like they were disappearing right out from under me. It was so sudden, astonishing and strange I didn't panic or get upset. I crawled to the side of the bed, pulled myself up and sat on the edge almost afraid to try again. Thinking if I gave my legs time perhaps they might go about doing what they had always done. I found that with concerted effort I could lift one leg at a time about an inch off the floor but couldn't place them with any control. Jen got up and came around to my side of the bed. "What's wrong?" I had no way of down-playing it. "I can't walk." "What!?" She sat down next to me and put her arm around my waist. "It's crazy but I can't get to my feet."

My balance and coordination had gone missing overnight. In an instant everything I was before: helpful, self reliant, strong, was gone. I had become helpless, dependent, weak. I needed Jen to help me dress and both her and our son Bluewolf to help me stand and support me as I shuffled from one clumsy numb foot to the other across the floor.

******

Growing up in the Midwest the idea of not pulling your own weight was a cardinal sin. I was proud and arrogant of my independence and the help I could offer others. When I saw someone in a wheelchair I felt pity for them but couldn't imagine accepting it for myself. I would rather be dead was what I felt at the time. If I can't be of use what's the use. This sense was bred into me by a busy-bee culture. Pull yourself up by your own bootstraps. God helps those who help themselves. We're even supposed to play hard. But helpless? For heaven's sake you better not be helpless. Helpless equals useless. But becoming helpless was one of the great lessons in life for me. It's what I was as a newborn but had long since forgotten. For it to happen again this time by a yet to be discovered cancerous tumor on my spine was a great humbler and perspective changer. From my helpless state I saw my family and friends spring into action. I was in awe of their generosity. The love and appreciation I felt for them has been one of the great gifts of my life. I've never seen a celestial angel but I've seen more than a few human angels.

****

My sudden inability to walk got me right in to see primary care physician, Dr. O'Kane, at UW Medicine clinic in Shoreline, Washington. Jen and Blue helped me down the fourteen steps of our suddenly daunting stairway—from the house to the driveway—and no handrail to hold on to. My legs were getting more numb by the hour. I could barely feel my feet. My right foot flopped around like a wet noodle it wouldn't plant flat on the ground. I also noticed a tight band of numbness around my midsection that felt like a belt cinched tight.

On the way to the clinic I thought of possible causes for my problem. I had been having painful muscle knots in my arms, neck and chest over the previous months and the last couple nights intense muscle spasms in my legs but felt no pain around my spine. I speculated that I slipped a disc while doing squats with weights or maybe it was from bending over and lifting a heavy box or perhaps I bumped into something I didn't remember. I thought of a lot of causes but a rapidly growing tumor on my spine was not one of them. I eat well, exercise regularly, don't smoke and rarely drink. Other than a tender elbow from chronic overuse, hay fever, and an occasional muscle pull, I've been healthy my entire adult life. I had no reason to believe it was anything life threatening. I was convinced that this was a fluke. Surely I tweaked something that only needed to be un-tweaked and then I could go about my life as usual.

At the clinic Jen retrieved a wheelchair while I struggled, braced against the car, up a short incline to the sidewalk and sat down hard in the wheelchair. She pushed me through the door for the first of what would become a mountain of medical appointments.

After an examination that included poking around on my legs, feet and midsection with a needle (I could feel the needle but it was dull) Dr. O'Kane looked concerned. She ordered a blood draw and a MRI of my lower spine to find or rule out the slipped disc that I insisted must be the cause of my lost balance and coordination. She also prescribed prednisone (a type of steroid) for the muscle pain I was experiencing. The steroid turned out to be a lucky turn because it happened to kill the type of cancer cells I didn't know I had. It likely retarded the growth of the tumor, saving me from more nerve damage. Sometimes luck in life cannot be overstated.

I was lucky again when Dr. O'Kane's assistant was able to get me the MRI appointment for later that day. I felt good about that. Waiting around for answers is not my strong suit. However, the quick appointment turned out to be a problem for our insurance coverage because they required several days for approval. I had to sign a promissory note that I was responsible for the full amount of around $5,000 if the insurance wasn't approved. I opted to sign the note. At least I would find out sooner what was wrong. It was the right choice, though at the time even the medical receptionist at the MRI center (as I was signing the paper) shook their head and lamented the ridiculous amount being charged for a forty-five minute scan. I found this sentiment to be true for almost everyone I encountered on my journey through the medical system. More than one doctor has described the obscene prices being charged for treating patients as criminal.

Inside the tube of the MRI machine I closed my eyes and submitted to an onslaught that was all encompassing. The technician had given me earplugs and headphones and a choice of music but they did little to stop an audio assault akin to a war zone, a construction site, and an alien invasion all happening at once. I kept my eyes closed, tried to breathe deep and slow, and looked forward to something good to eat when I was out of there.

It was sinking in that the fix for this mess would involve spinal surgery and all the uncertainties that came along with it. It doesn't do any good to speculate. I'm zero for whatever vs the infinitely variable universe. Still, it's so damn hard not to wonder what's next? And when it looks bad start imagining the worst.

Back home, late afternoon, in bed, I tried to downplay my predicament in my mind. Yes, I was in my mid-fifties and it was stupid to be doing over-zealous workouts at my age. When Dr. O'Kane sees the slipped disc on the MRI I'll be under doctor's orders to go easy from here on out. Maybe I'll listen then. I never knew when to stop. I had a gimpy elbow because I wouldn't stop playing the guitar when it started to hurt. Instead, I pushed it beyond its limit and now I had done the same to my back. It seemed I would never learn. I wiggled my numb toes and sighed. Yeah this will teach me.

Dr. O'Kane called the next morning (Friday the 13th). The MRI of my lower back hadn't revealed a slipped disc but there was something about my blood that wasn't right and did I know I was anemic? I didn't. She requested a larger blood sample and wanted me to come in right away. "What is it?" I asked, thinking this is out of left field. She wasn't ready to confirm anything but would let me know as soon as she got a look at another blood sample. That's just the thing that can get my mind going. First I thought it was a mistake, I felt all right—a hell of a con given I was unable to walk on my own, could barely sit up in bed, and apparently I was anemic. Then my mind went the other way, this was bad, what was I thinking, I can't walk, of course this was bad. Then back, there's nothing to worry about it's something simple maybe the MRI missed some nerve damage. The slipped disc might be further up my spine. It had to be there what else could it be? That night I spoke about it with Jen and we concluded that it was likely something small that had been overlooked. There was no need to overthink it. I would be okay.

Saturday morning I went back to the clinic to give more blood. As before Jen retrieved a wheelchair, I labored up the little slope, sat down, and she pushed me inside. In addition to the blood they wanted a urine sample. An hour later I was back home in bed wondering why all the blood? What did it have to do with a slipped disc?

I struggled through the weekend forced to recon with my limitations. Jen found an old cane in a closet that I had used as a prop in a short film. With the cane on one side and a wall on the other I could shuffle slowly through the house. It was a shock to find that shuffling from the bedroom to the kitchen and back left me breathing hard. Taking a shower was out the question. Instead, I slumped down in the tub, white steam rising to meet the dark cloud over my head. Getting in and out of the tub was a hazard. Almost everything was a hazard. I did a lot of crawling. All the little things I took for granted, like dressing, became slow and tedious. Even turning over in bed was an effort. I tried to keep a positive outlook. I would be calm in the assurance that everything is temporary including this, then I would chastise myself again for attempting squats with weights and messing up my back. That's the problem with aging, your body gets older but your mind stays the same. If it wasn't for the mirror I would swear

I was still in my twenties. That's what I was doing, exercising like I was still in my twenties.

Tuesday, midmorning, Dr. O'Kane called and I could tell by her tone it wasn't good. After a short back and forth she shook me with, "Your bone marrow is spitting out malignant cells," then sent my head reeling with, "it looks like cancer." She said something about a Seattle Cancer Care Alliance and would send a referral right away. What? Slow down this is too fast. The word cancer blotted out everything all I could see was 'CANCER' in all caps and bold black letters. Had I been able to stand the news would have sent me staggering. "They'll call you to setup an appointment." I was only half listening. My mind was racing with, cancer in the bloodstream, cancer in the bloodstream, cancer in the bloodstream, that means it's everywhere in my body, cancer in the bloodstream, cancer in the bloodstream, from what I know it's a sure killer. I blurted out, "This sounds like a death sentence." There was pause on the other end. I don't think she was expecting me to be so matter of fact. She said, "I'm sorry to give you the bad news." I thanked her and hung up the phone. My slipped disc scenario slipped out of sight with this horrifying turn of events. I was dying.

****

Cancer comes with a sudden confrontation with death. My mortality was now front and center. I found myself in this position for the first time. The word alone squeezed my heart, put a pit in my stomach, vertigo in my head, and shook my numb and nearly useless legs. I knew cancer was a prevailing threat for young and old but until it hits close to home its abstract and elsewhere. It took a sledgehammer to my life and left me dazed. Nothing looked the same after hearing that word. I clung to what little hope I could conjure up in my mind that maybe it was a mistake and further tests might confirm that it was something else. I wanted so much to get up, pace the floor, and think about it, outrun it if I had to, but not be stuck in bed. The little hope I was clinging to quickly faded. I wasn't one to bullshit myself when a situation revealed itself to be something I didn't like. My sudden paralysis wasn't as simple as I had made it out to be. The dread I felt thinking I would have to endure back surgery was mild in comparison to what I felt now. Something else was going on and it was happening to me. Still, I was thankful it was me and not my wife or children. I couldn't bear it if this was happening to one of them.

12

Life is about change and it is the same for us. Yet we avoid change because its inconvenient, unknown, uncertain, attached to our fears and vulnerabilities. This avoidance is powerful and stops us from ending bad habits, seeking deeper love and appreciation for life, our family, community, other nations, other folks who share this miracle stone we call home. Given a choice we lean toward the same old comforts. The proliferation of objects invented to make life more comfortable confirms this. In our comfort we fall into routines and life tends to grey and blend together. Time speeds up. Blank days fan out behind us. Change arrives in the form of a confrontation. Confrontations wake us up. Cancer is one hell of a confrontation and man did it wake me up! Sometimes when we're in a confrontation the quality of our response is terrible and we go along kicking and screaming about our situation but often times later on we come to regard it as positive and even necessary for our growth and the new opportunities that resulted.

There is a logic behind going for the best quality response when facing a major confrontation because we don't know what the outcome will be in advance. Prejudging any situation is a mistake. Sometimes it takes years to discover whether an event from the past has turned out good or bad. This is difficult to do especially in a culture that is full of judgment. Everyone it seems is eager to tell us what is good and what is bad. "Too soon to tell" might be worth repeating to ourselves when we're faced with a confrontation. I'm convinced that the folks I've witnessed having poor responses to their challenges conjured up more difficulties along the way.

****

I knew Jen would be calling later in the morning to check in and find out if I had heard from the doctor. I resolved that when she called I wasn't going to tell her what Dr. O'Kane had told me. It would be better to tell her at home.

I laid in bed feeling perplexed but with the growing realization that the doctor would not have said cancer if she hadn't seen ample proof. She couldn't give me a definitive diagnosis but I knew she had found the source of my issues and that I had to accept it. I was dying. I didn't think it would happen like this but then again who does. I didn't feel self-pity or resentment. I've thought about death many times over the years the sheer inevitability of it made it a subject for serious consideration. We're all going to die. I'm not sure how anyone can ignore it. We all know its coming and there is no avoiding it but it is something few want to talk or even think about. We shun it like the devil. Death remains unresolved. It is a subject we must work out individually despite the taboo. It backfires on those who don't get around to it when cancer or some other calamity comes along and all they can do is look away or deny it's happening. Though I have con-templated death over the years, it is one thing to think about something, but another to be facing it.

When Jen called and asked if I had heard anything from Dr. O'Kane my resolve not to tell her until she got home quickly dissipated. Though I tried I wasn't used to hiding things from her. I said, "No," took a breath then said, "yes, the doctor told me there is cancer in my blood." She left work. We had a whole new reality to deal with. It's a blessing to have such an amazing partner in life but in a sudden situation of vulnerability and need the blessing reveals itself in full bloom. I can't give her enough credit for getting us through this extremely difficult journey. Cancer reveals if you have partnered well and whether you treated those in your life with love and respect. Later when I was prepping for a bone marrow transplant I met a man in the waiting area who said his wife refused to make the long drive with him for his treatments. He was alone and I wondered whether he married poorly or had been a selfish husband whose partner had finally had enough. Even her husband's cancer didn't move her to stand beside him. He was on his own through what was likely the most difficult journey of his life and had no one to hold his hand and tell him he was loved.

That afternoon I got a call from a scheduler at Seattle Cancer Care Alliance (SCCA). The next available appointment was the morning of Monday, April 23, six days away. Six days felt like a long time to wait. I assumed my rapidly declining health constituted an emergency so given it was almost a week before I would be seen it was because either it wasn't an emergency or I was already so far gone it didn't matter. It might be a pitstop on the way to hospice. Maybe they were being considerate giving me the week to get my affairs in order. My mind was so muddled I didn't consider the obvious

—that there were other folks out there dealing with cancers of their own who were in or entering the system just like me. I couldn't expect to jump ahead of them.

There wasn't much to get in order regarding my affairs. As a DIY musician/writer I've had a precious life of freedom and fulfillment though not much in the way of money and things. I hadn't put off till later what I could do right then and that's probably the source of my lack of self-pity and resentments. I was never working for retirement or waiting to pursue my interests. I was satisfied to leave behind a few books, poems, essays and a couple hundred songs spread over twenty-something records. Honestly, it didn't mean that much to me anymore. My family was the big prize and I wanted to give them everything I had for as long as I had left.

Later in the day we told our son about my cancer. His face twisted in pain and his eyes squeezed tight as he said, "I'm not ready to lose my dad." It broke my heart to see him in such anguish. I tried to console him, offering that he was ready for whatever came his way and besides we didn't know what my cancer entailed so it was best to wait and see. Easy to say to him not so easy to do for myself. The next day in an absurd attempt at some last minute instruction I had him help me to the car so I could show him again how to check the oil, refill the coolant, position the jack, change a tire. Looking back I don't think he was even listening. His dad was dying.

My son Bluewolf is a when-the-chips-are-down type of person. Indeed, he fits his unusual name (a combination of name and place from both sides of his family) You can't get him to pick up after himself (a symptom of his young age) but if it's important he will carry you into next week. I experienced this quality when he was fifteen and we went to see his granddad, my dad, on his death bed. When I saw my dad I fully realized all the softness that laid beneath his hardshell that never allowed intimacy or anything real and honest between us. I felt a surge of guilt for never having broken through. I was an emotional yoyo for the rest of the visit while my son rode with me, crying when I cried, but then interjecting with some wise insight like, "He can't show how he really feels but you know it's there," or, "it wasn't your job to fix him," that shifted the mood from loss to introspection. Steadfast and true he carried me through the experience.

We had to tell our daughter Ocean (another name given in inspiration) living in New York about my cancer over the phone. She knew something was up when she got a text telling her to call home. Right off the bat she was adamant that this was not as bad as it seemed saying, "You're one of the strongest people I know, dad. I just know that you'll get through this okay." She buoyed us with daily texts and calls and FaceTime. She was a positive force during our week of uncertainty, refusing to believe this was the end of her dad. Her positivity was much needed and it turned out she was correct I'm still here.

On Thursday, April 19, I received a packet of information from SCCA. Seeing my name on a large envelope from a cancer institute felt strange and unsettling. It was one hell of a reality shift. I gave the packet a loose looking at. It confirmed my appointment on the 23rd with a team led by oncologist Dr. Cowan. According to the information SCCA was a collaboration between Fred Hutchinson Cancer Research, Children's Hospital, and University of Washington Medicine. There was an 8 1/2 by 11 inch ring bound patient care manual that contained one hundred and fifty-three pages. I flipped through the pages from back to front stopping only once. I caught a glimpse of the glossary of terms and a short section titled What's Next? I held up in the Coping with Symptoms chapter when I saw pictures of food. Under the title: Diet Guidelines for Immunosuppressed Patients were foods that could be eaten and others that could not. It was bad news for sushi lovers. I continued on flipping past pages titled White Blood Cells, Sexuality, Peripheral Neuropathy, Memory and Concentration, Dehydration, and through the Getting Started chapter to the front cover then slid the manual back into the large envelope and set it aside. I just didn't have an appetite for it. I liked the world I was in before this. I wasn't ready for this new one written in black and white.

The days dragged on and it felt like I was in limbo. I had cancer in my blood but which one? I knew of someone who had leukemia when I was young and it killed them awfully quick. I made the choice not to search online because the internet tends to be full of worst case scenarios and I didn't want to be influenced by expectations and the experiences of others. I didn't want to confirm what I felt— that this was the worst thing ever.

My speculating mind was my biggest obstacle with its constant projecting of what ifs: What if I never walk again? What if I die sooner than later? What if it gets more painful? My mind can easily make what ifs into concrete platforms on which to stand and lament. All this speculation and worry was energy draining and pointless because we can never know what's in store for us tomorrow. I didn't need any more fuel for the fear from the internet. Looking back now it was the right choice for me. Another solid reason I discovered later was the extreme range of results patients have with their cancer and treatments. It runs the gamut between a benign tumor and hospice two weeks after diagnosis. It is never the same. Even the same cancer affects everyone differently even as the same treatments are being applied. There are so many variables at work depending on the advance of the disease, physical health, age, outlook, the list goes on. It's easy to get ahead of yourself and get pinned down by expectations. It's also true that everyone reacts to their situation differently. I would discover a few more times before I was through that no matter what is occurring everyone has a choice how to respond and those I saw who accepted their reality with positivity did much better than those who did not.

In many ways cancer is a truth serum. In its extremity it reveals a person's character in full. Sitting in the waiting areas for my appointments (over the course of my treatments this amounted to many hours) it was easy to see those who were suffering over their suffering, i.e., those who had a bad case of the why-me's. I watched them squirming in their seats, scowling at their cell phones, looking up abruptly and scanning the room with a bitter look. Still, we were all there hoping to go on living in whatever form we were already existing.

I was spending so much time in bed each day my glutes knotted up making it all but impossible to sit or lie down without extreme discomfort. By Friday, April 20, I was so desperate I called my clinic to see if I could get a couple injections of muscle relaxers, anything to relieve the pain, but was told it wouldn't do any good. I took it in the worse way, of course it wouldn't do any good I was done for. It was apparent that I didn't have long to live. I was deteriorating so rapidly there was no way to slow it down. To think I was hiking only a month before and now I was anemic, gaunt, grey and bedridden. Without regular movement and exercise my legs were atrophying by the day. My strength was slipping away. When our daughter called to say she was flying home in three weeks I thought that might be too late and wondered if I should insist she fly home sooner. Considering how quickly my body was failing me at this rate three weeks seemed so far away. There was no telling the state I would be in by then. I didn't want her to arrive when I was choking on my last breath unable to say goodbye, I love you.

As the week wore on, my speculating mind rampaged with worst-case scenarios. The stress was getting to me. I tried to remain calm by breathing deep and reminding myself again I didn't know what the future held. Ten minutes later I was back in my speculating mind dramatizing the future.

With my cane, a wall to steady myself, and a force of will I didn't know I had in me I moved slowly from room to room. I had accumulated piles of music and written material over the years. They were spread throughout the house in boxes and drawers and closets. So many unfinished projects that I didn't wan't to burden my family with after I was gone. I sorted through and threw away most of them—torn in half and ready for recycling. I was glad to have this busy work to occupy myself even though I could only work fifteen minutes at a time before needing to rest. Sometimes as I rested I reflected on my life. All the ups and downs. The weaving course my life had taken. It astonished me that I had arrived at such a good place with a family I loved dearly and who loved me the same. In so many ways it appeared that I had blundered into it only half aware of what I was doing and where I was going. It's the serendipitous nature of life that makes it appear that so many important outcomes turned on the smallest moments and changed the direction of my life so completely for the better.

****

I was shaped both bad and good by my dad. He saw the world as essentially corrupt so he moved the family to an old homestead in northern Minnesota in the early seventies. Unable to support a family of five on twenty acres he held a day job in the nearby town while mom, my two sisters, but mostly me, were left to work the farm.

As the only son I carried the burden of his expectations and being a sensitive kid I had trouble carrying on the role of the tough country boy he expected. Growing up under his all-controlling overbearing personality set me in search of a life of rich diversion as a counterbalance. When I wasn't in my head leaping tall buildings or saving damsels in distress I was in pursuit of lake superior agates, filling coffee cans and dreaming of more, or four leaf clovers, collecting thousands and pressing them between the pages of our encyclopedias, when someone opened a volume flattened four leaf clovers fell out everywhere.

Languishing under my dad's rule I developed a staunch resistance to authority that continued into adulthood. Sometimes for the better but other times not. I left a lot of good advice from well-meaning people on the table, mistaking their good intentions for bad authority. The other damage my dad inflicted was by continually shaming me. I had a natural enthusiasm for life and a tendency to jump around and get excited about anything out of the ordinary. In those moments he would insult, ridicule, and belittle me, often in front of other people. I learned to keep my enthusiasms away from his presence. But it was deeply hurtful.

It was my mom who bore witness to my dad's behavior and made it a point to assure me many times over that it was him, not me, who was the problem. However, in the fashion of someone who grew up with an alcoholic dad (she was as abused as I was) she avoided confrontation with her husband. I was begged to apologize for whatever he did so there would be peace. The injustice of that really sank in deep, and consequently as an adult it is still the injustices in the world that get to me the most.

It's the shaming that is the most difficult to overcome. All slights are exaggerated for those shamed in childhood. Shame is a poison in the mind that takes years to dilute. My reckless years from fifteen to twenty-four, of alcohol, drugs, and outlandish behavior, were wanton acts of self destruction fueled by the shame heaped on me as a kid. Discovering the guitar, writing and singing, helped me turn the poison into medicine. But the most profound impact on my healing came from a choice I made in my late twenties. We've all heard the phrase "we don't pick our parents". I've said it myself on occasion when complaining about my dad and the lack of love and encouragement I received growing up. But there is a futility to this statement that always bothered me. So I decided to take the position that I did choose my parents. It sounds absurd but what it did was take me from a passive role to an active one. It put me in a more powerful position. I was no longer a leaf being blown on the winds of chance. An unlucky soul who through happenstance got an unlucky start. The choice that I picked my parents did wonders for my spiritual and emotional healing. It was because I didn't need my dad to make amends, accept responsibility and make it right, which he could never do. All my childhood experiences shifted from passive victimhood to active obstacles that had readied me for my life ahead. Indeed, the good things that I had forgotten from my youth, which I had shuttered away in my misery, came to the forefront and I could better see that it hadn't been all bad. The work I endured on the farm built up a discipline in me that contributed greatly to my ability to persevere through the doubt and uncertainty of being a musician and writer. I was able to take risks and enter new territory musically. This required a thick skin when critics came to knock me around. I could be absurd in my art at times because life itself is absurd. It's the strangest thing to be alive. I imagine it will be strange to be dead. I've turned away from the modern view that we are just tiny little specks in the face of an immense universe. It strikes me as pathetic and full of false humility. How humble are people who are busy converting the infinite natural world into a finite material world? Here as well I made the active choice considering perhaps it took a universe of this enormity to manifest life. Life that could then evolve and look upon itself with awe and wonder. And we chose it all.

****

By Saturday, April 21, I was really struggling. The prednisone I was taking kept me awake and wiped me out. My sleep deprived weary mind saw a future short and bleak and there was nothing I could do about it. My usual way to reduce worry and stress had always been to get moving, go for a hike or whatever, but there I was tethered to my bed. My body was in ruins and I could only lie there wrought with uncertainty and speculation. It was nearly impossible to keep my mind from going to those awful places that a tired, worried head is bound to fly off to. It was getting the better of me throughout the day, and then in the early evening, alone in bed, feeling so down and beat, I got the notion that I would die right then and there. Yes, I was dying right there. In the stress of the moment I stopped breathing and became lightheaded which induced me to believe it even more. I wanted so much to leap out of bed and run for the door. I called out to Jen in my fright, but when she came into the bedroom and asked what was wrong, in my lowballing midwestern way I choked out, "I'm not feeling so good." There I was thinking I was on death's door and I was underplaying it! Jen saw that I was panicking. I was as white as a ghost. She laid down in bed next to me, held my hand and said, "It's going to be okay just breathe." I took big heaving gulps of air and exhaled toward the ceiling. My lightheadedness passed. I wasn't dying just then. We held hands lying next to each other in bed. I stared up at the ceiling feeling so stupid, thinking how ridiculous I was, and how easy it was to get hung up in fear and panic. A moment later the words Love, Trust, Gratitude, and Healing floated into my head. I latched onto them repeating, Love, Trust, Gratitude, Healing, Love, Trust, Gratitude, Healing. A calmness enveloped me. These were words worth meditating on and repeating. Even the order of them struck me as meaningful.

That night I had a dream. Death entered my room, more shadow than substance, leaned over me and said, "Breathe this in if you can. Life and I are partners. We cannot be separated. Being in Life you're prejudiced against me. But I give Life meaning." I awoke with a start. Death was gone. I stared at the dark ceiling and thought about the dream. It was true, Life I knew and loved. I clung to it. Death was unknown and scary. But if Life and Death make a whole, then it's a mistake to separate them and value one over the other. It makes sense that we should thank death for life. When someone commits suicide we say it was because they couldn't handle life. But maybe we say this because we can't handle death. It dawned on me that desiring to live on and on was a naive wish. It's naive because it would spell the end of life as the vital all-important event we all experience. We know we're alive in relation to knowing we will be dead someday. We see this truth in our stories of vampires who live forever only by sucking the life out of the living and must remain in the dark. They so long for death they sleep in coffins, yet they're still afraid to die. These stories are cultural mirrors that express the folly of desiring to live forever. Let's dispel the notion that life and death are separate. Therefore, fear of death is fear of life.

Cancer brought me face to face with my death but also with my life. It shredded all my plans and machinations and when they were lying there scattered in front of me, essentially worthless, I realized I had been mostly paying attention to the surface of things. Cancer forced me inside of myself. I assumed death would arrive from out there somewhere but here it was taking me from the inside. Going forward I felt that the challenge I was facing with cancer and my uncertain future was to remain open and curious, not closed off and fearful. When I caught myself speculating in fear I repeated Love Trust Gratitude Healing and it helped me remain present, open and curious—not all—but most of the time.

It's true I'm going to die and with cancer the process may have accelerated but I don't want to be desperate about staying alive. It's also true when I first heard my doctor say cancer I never wanted to live more. Not just to live but to live more meaningfully. Eyes wide open! I was reawakened to what is and has always been important. I saw my life and those in it and I wanted more of them. Yes, cancer stripped away the hubris in my life: status, accomplishments, ego driven goals. All those important things I have since forgotten.

I slept a few hours after the dream and woke up Sunday morning feeling much better. I continued to think about my dream and the truth of it. Monday I would find out what ailed me and what options I had going forward. If it was death sooner than later I would have to accept it.

****

On Monday, Jen and I arrived at SCCA for my 9:00 a.m. appointment heavy with anticipation. We parked on level A beneath the building. My legs were shot but I had an overwhelming desire to walk to my appointment. Call it Irish pride, I don't know, but I was determined not to use a wheelchair. I wanted to meet my destiny standing on my feet. I walked slowly, leaning on my cane, holding Jen's hand for balance, trying not to convey the tremendous effort it took to get from the car to the elevator, the elevator to registration on the first floor. I got a much needed break sitting for a few minutes while they gathered my information. Then it was on to another set of elevators and up to the fourth floor (Hematology Oncology) check in and waiting area. Luckily the layout of the building was compact, otherwise I wouldn't have made it.

The waiting area had large windows and comfortable chairs. We'd just sat down when my name was called mistakenly pronounced Mc-Death which turned a few heads as Jen stood up, helped me up and we prepared to follow the nurse who asked, "Did I pronounce that right?" "No, it's pronounced Mc-Day-eth." "Oh, I'm sorry." "No problem, everybody does it."
She led us to an examination room where we waited for Dr. Cowan who arrived a few minutes later followed by his Clinical Nurse Coordinator Ryan and Physician Assistant Lauren.

We liked Dr. Cowan right away. He seemed open and honest and told us straight away that I had a cancer called multiple myeloma. The bad news—it was incurable. The good news—it was treatable with ninety percent of patients living five years and fifty percent living ten years or more. Thirty years ago cancers like multiple myeloma were sure killers but thanks to Dr. E. Donnall Thomas and his team working at Fred Hutchinson Cancer Research Center here in Seattle innovative techniques were developed and patient's lives have been extended with some people surviving decades. I hope to be one of them. Jen and I were holding hands at the time and we nearly squeezed the blood out of our fingers when we heard my passing wasn't imminent. I had an excellent chance of making it at least five years or longer. Compared to the five weeks I thought I had left, hearing I may have five years felt like a lifetime. I cannot express the joy and utter relief we felt that it wasn't terminal. It gave us an energy that snapped and crackled. I suspect this is true for many as it was for me that after the shock of diagnoses I never wanted to live more. It's odd to consider that cancer brings an acuity for life. A life with renewed appreciation, a vigor perhaps hidden beneath routine and all the little details that distract us moment by moment. It was palpable and it went on for several weeks during which time strangers would come up to us and just start talking. One day when we were waiting for an appointment, holding hands as usual, a woman came over to us and spontaneously put her hands over our hands, smiled and said, "I don't know what this is about but I feel like I want to be a part of it." We laughed and said, "Of course you can."

Dr. Cowan went on to outline possible treatments and which ones he thought would be the most effective for me culminating with a bone marrow transplant. None of it would be easy, especially the transplant. I would do the heavy lifting. Truthfully, I was hardly listening to him. It was much like when I heard Dr. O'Kane say the word cancer, and I could only think, I'm going to die! Now I could only think, I'm going to live! The physical sensations were identical: it squeezed my heart, put a pit in my stomach, vertigo in my head, and shook my numb and nearly useless legs.

Toward the end of our appointment, as Dr. Cowan was entering information on the computer, a hummingbird appeared at the window and bumped against the glass as though trying to get in. Hummingbirds have always been a favorite of mine. The window looks out on the I-5 corridor as it passes through downtown Seattle. With a mountain of grey concrete as a backdrop a hummingbird looked wildly out of place. When we pointed it out Dr. Cowan said, "That's a good sign." Jen and I heartily agreed. If nothing else it was a beautiful life affirming sight. Yes, I would like to see more of that.

I got yet another lucky turn when his assistant Lauren suggested that the reason for my loss of balance and coordination might be due to spinal cord compression from a tumor. She had worked with a spinal surgeon for a number of years and knew the telltale signs. Dr. Cowan immediately ordered an MRI scan for my entire spine. After a few more details he sent us to see his team coordinator, Michael, who heroically got us a MRI appointment for early that afternoon. He was able to get the appointment even though, again, the insurance wasn't approved. It was the second time in ten days we were required to sign a paper stating we were responsible for the full amount—this time something like sixteen thousand dollars. We were already over twenty-thousand dollars in debt for just two MRIs. These fees really are ridiculous, whether we had to pay them or an insurance company for that matter. My insurance company did end up paying for both MRI's once they had been established as a cancer related emergency.

We had a couple hours before my MRI appointment, so instead of going home we got lunch then drove to Gas Works Park located on the north shore of Lake Union. It was warm for April. We found a spot in the shade and sat on the grass. Gas Works Park is a special place for us because we got married there in the nineties. We had a sunrise ceremony on the sundial at the top of the knoll. It had been an incredible start to our wedding day with a beautiful sunrise in the East while lightning flashed and thunder clapped to the South and a rainbow stretched between Queen Anne hill and the Fremont neighborhood. It was an incredible scene and a great memory, but now I couldn't climb the knoll to the sundial.

I spent an hour and a half in the MRI tube. Afterward we drove home and we were there less than twenty minutes when Dr. Cowan called and said they had found the cause of my loss of balance and coordination. There was a tumor over-lapping my T5 and T6 vertebrae (middle back corresponding with the numbness that I felt around my midsection) compressing my spinal cord. Multiple myeloma cells love bone. Once they escape the bloodstream and attach them-selves to bone they begin to reproduce exponentially thus explaining my sudden loss of balance and coordination. We were to immediately go to the emergency room at the University of Washington Medical Center.

****

I needed all the elation and adrenaline flow for the emergency room that I got from the news my cancer was treatable. We sat in a cramped waiting area squeezed by a construction project going on around us but we were not bothered at all. We continued to bask in the good news we'd received. We were practically pinching ourselves and each other. It was a shower of relief after the long uncertain week we endured, Jen, picking up the slack after I clattered to the floor, keeping herself upright and positive through her own sleepless nights. And me, hoping to live, preparing to die, the whole up and down, will I, won't I, turmoil of it. Now as I sat waiting for Mc-Death to be called out it entered my head—did I throw away that book I had nearly finished writing when I was discarding my projects? I hoped not. I was already making plans for the future though now it was a five year plan. Time was truly of the essence.

The good news released a pressure cooker inside me and I exploded with love in every direction. It was like the last door to my heart blew open and I couldn't help myself. I blessed everyone who entered my view—wishing for them great health and long life. If I sensed that they were suffering I blessed them twice. I thought of Love Trust Gratitude Healing (LTGH). Suddenly I realized that I had been repeating an equation or a recipe. As a recipe: Love, Trust and

Gratitude are the ingredients and Healing is the result. As an equation: Love + Trust + Gratitude = Healing. It made sense. Love begets Trust, Trust begets Gratitude and with all three there is Healing. In the middle of this revelation I heard the call, "Michael Mc-Death."

I spent about eight hours in ER telling my story, answering the same questions and going through the same tests for measuring my leg and arm strength. I lifted, pressed, pushed and resisted upon request. Several times I was instructed to roll on my side and squeeze down as hard as possible when a gloved finger was inserted into my rectum. This was no time for vanity, I said to myself. I would say it a few mores times before I was finished with my cancer treatments.

I repeated my story to at least a half dozen spinal and neurological doctors who listened attentively then ran me through the motor skill tests. UW Medical Center is attached to the University of Washington and therefore is a learning institution so medical students abounded. It seemed every one of them paid me a visit, asking to hear my story and going through the testing routine. There was so much interest it seemed like I was the curious case of Michael McDaeth.

Between visits from nurses, doctors, and interns, Jen and I continued to talk about the relief we felt after our meeting with Dr. Cowan. Hearing that some had been living normal lives for decades with the disease gave us hope that maybe I might make it a good stretch. I declared that my goal was thirty years. Outrageous but why not? We mapped out the coming weeks, the time off she would need to take for appointments and when I was going through the bone marrow transplant. We talked about the people we needed to tell about my cancer.

****

I noticed two common reactions from people when they were told I had cancer. The larger percentage reacted with concern, sadness and pity. They asked how I was doing, said unconvincingly that I was looking good, inquired about the treatments, nodded their heads with sad pressed lips. The smaller percentage didn't want to linger on the subject at all. It's as if they feared it might rub off on them just by talking about it. When they heard the word cancer they turned their heads as though it had given them a glancing blow. Cancer is the bogeyman of death. I found these encounters awkward and uncomfortable and when possible tried to communicate that I didn't feel this was as tragic a situation as it could have been. I had thought I would be gone in a matter of weeks. I had some breathing room. The world sparkled and the street had an other-worldly shine. There's no escaping it—we're all going to die. It's just easier to ignore when one is healthy. I wanted to tell everyone who gave the pity-look that there was more to this than meets the eye. I was awake and my heart had expanded tenfold. The few I told continued to nod their heads out of habit but with an expression that conveyed they thought I was nuts. Like the only prize in life was to go on living hassle-free.

****

There was considerable debate between Neurology and Radiation Oncology whether to remove the tumor by surgery or use radiation to deal with it. I was told at one point that it would be up to me to decide. I found this stressful. I hadn't the slightest clue which was the better option. Would someone from each department present their case with a pointer and an x-ray of my tumored spine, give assessments, the risks involved, length of recovery?

After the first few hectic hours the traffic to my bedside dropped off. As more hours ticked away Jen and I were left wondering what was causing the delay. I found out later that all the action was happening behind the scenes. Information was moving up and down the chain of command of the two separate departments. Eventually it was verified that the tumor was from the multiple myeloma and a doctor from Radiation Oncology explained the course was now clear. Radiation was the better option as it was effective at killing multiple myeloma cells. Around two in the morning I was moved to the seventh floor cancer ward. I would begin radiation treatments later that day.

I didn't get much sleep. So much had transpired in such a short time that my mind whirled, plus I find hospital beds really uncomfortable. I raised and lowered the head, foot and middle trying to find a position that didn't make my body ache. Around six in the morning a nurse arrived to give me pills in little paper cups and a shot in the belly. Later I ordered breakfast—a spinach frittata—it wasn't bad. By mid afternoon I was in a wheelchair on my way to Radiation Oncology, pushed along by a volunteer (a medical undergrad) for the first of ten radiation treatments to deal with the tumor on my spine. We rolled down look-a-like hallways to an elevator and descended to the basement where I was pushed through the automatic sliding glass doors of Radiation Oncology into line at reception.

The waiting area was packed. We were all there to get lit up by one of the radiation machines. We arrived from everywhere, all walks of life, rich, poor, black, white—cancer exempted no one. We had become sisters and brothers now, though I'm inclined to think that had always been true but it took something like this for us to recognize it. Some of us arrived alone, a few like myself in wheelchairs, others on crutches, a number with an entourage where one could easily pick out the patient. Most showed up with a partner, a wife, a husband, sometimes a brother or sister, an adult child. All of us were there to face our fears.

Over the course of my treatments I found Radiation Oncology to have the most intense waiting area. Perhaps because many patients were in a more acute condition or maybe it's just the aspect of receiving a blast of radiation that doesn't settle well in our minds. The mood was heavy. There was a woman who wore her cancer on her face, she couldn't close her mouth, cancer occupied her jaw. I had the feeling she might be as distraught over the visible effects as the cancer itself. I felt bad for her and wished her love and peace of mind. There was a man sitting alone on the opposite side of the room who kept smiling, giggling, and nodding his head at me but not in a kind way—more like he was taking some sinister pleasure in us being there together. I wasn't sure what to make of him but it did seem his situation was pushing him over the edge. When his name was called he struggled to his feet by hoisting himself up on a pair of crutches then twisting his hips to throw his feet forward, he lurched awkwardly out of the waiting area. He wasn't much more than a collection of bones under a drapery of clothes. I wanted to jump out of my wheelchair, run over and give him a hug, and wish him a mountain of luck and love.

As I mentioned I had an overwhelming impulse to love on everyone with whom I crossed paths. Maybe because I knew the end had shrunk for me so what was I waiting for?

I've always had a sense for people in pain but kept it to myself most of the time because I'm not a naturally outgoing person. I assumed everyone preferred to be left alone, but what I've found in the last year is the need people have for real connection. Cancer turns everything on its head. It's a good place to bridge the gaps between us. It might be that in conjunction with great loss comes a new openness of being. After having exceptional health my entire life, here I was barely able to move but I was okay—physically I was a wreck but emotionally and spiritually I was really okay. I had enough in me to give whatever I could to others who were suffering.

When it was my turn a nurse appeared and wheeled me past reception, through a door, past examination rooms, and radiation machines, to a changing area with curtained booths and lockers where I stripped down and put on a hospital gown. Leaning heavily on my cane I made my way past the radiation machine control booth, through a vault-like opening, with its thick lead-lined door swung wide. I moved into a large space where I was helped by two friendly technicians to lie down on the table under the radiation machine. They carefully nudged me into position. One of them said that this would be my longest appointment because they had to establish the location the radiation beam would strike the tumor. When I was in the right spot they drew a target on my chest and tattooed in permanent ink a couple freckle-sized marks on both sides of my ribcage so they could easily triangulate the exact location for each radiation treatment. A cushion was tucked under my head. It reminded me of styrofoam except it was pliable and they shaped it to best support and keep my head in place. They wrote my name on it and after each session it was hung on a clothes rack with dozens of others to await my return. When they were ready I was instructed to grab hold of two metal pegs that jutted out above my head to keep my arms out of the way while the machine was operating. In the few seconds it took for the technicians to vacate the room, close the thick lead-lined door, and start the machine, I thanked the multiple myeloma for the lessons and insights I was gaining—then politely asked it to go away. I did this before all ten of my radiation treatments. I had decided to make peace with my cancer instead of considering it my enemy because intuitively I felt that relaxation, acceptance, and calmness were the states of being that would give me the best chance for optimal recovery. With tension, pain increases and immunity suffers.

I've noticed over the course of my life that whenever I've been really stressed out or emotionally down inevitably I got sick. Stress and immunity are not friends.

The radiation treatment involved the machine firing a radiation beam at the tumor from above before rotating under table and shooting a beam from below. It was over in seconds and it felt like nothing happened. The thick lead-lined door opened, the technicians entered, helped me off the table, and handed me my cane. I made my way to the dressing room for my clothes then to the wheelchair and back to the reception area. I waited until another volunteer arrived and wheeled me to my room till the next day when we repeated the routine.

After the third radiation treatment I was released from the hospital and I finished as an outpatient with Jen driving us to the hospital, retrieving a wheelchair and pushing me to Radiation Oncology.

There's a small gong on the wall in the reception area. Folks who have completed all their radiation treatments bang the gong as they are leaving for the last time and everybody applauds. Sometimes they're compelled to say a few words to encourage the rest of us. It raises everyone's spirits and for a few moments we are one in our experiences. Eyes meet and smiles are shared. Sometimes conversations are struck up and time glides along easily. Eventually we return to our personal experience and private suffering.

I was put on a 40 mg daily dose of dexamethasone in the form of ten tiny white pills to go along with the radiation. Dexamethasone is a powerful steroid combined with a strong stimulant. It may be effective for killing multiple myeloma cells but not for sleep. I seldom slept more than an hour or two at a time. The drug just kept me whistling along. I was also taking an anti-seizure medication. During this stretch of time I found myself up at night, bent on solving the world's problems. I equated my tumor to a tumor on the spine of the nation, keeping the good people broke from profiteering corporations and an incompetent corrupt government. I could see clearly that the truth must be told and it was up to me to do so. I planned on doing a podcast, writing books, starting a national campaign to bring about the changes that were needed. I saw myself as the only one capable of bringing the truth to the world. I was so pumped up with energy and conviction and no sleep I believed I could and would do it all. After a few nights of over-the-top mental campaigning I happened to read the side effects of the anti-seizure medication. One of the first listed was delusions of grandeur. I laughed, man did I have that! Combined with the daily dose of dexamethasone it must have dialed up a few notches. Every so often I had to remind myself that it was the meds talking.

I was still on dexamethasone when I met with my radiologist, Dr. Tseng, for the first time and when she saw the daily dose of 40 mg on my chart her eyes widened with concern. She commented that it was a strong dose and I shouldn't be taking that much every day. A plan was implemented to wean me off the drug by reducing the dose by one pill per day over an eight day period. This turned out to be one of the more difficult things to get through. In the short time of taking it I had become dependent. Each reduction brought aniexty, muscle tension and clenched teeth. I had trouble following through with the plan. At 12 mg I had to go with a smaller reduction because of the awful aniexty I was feeling. By the end I was cutting the last couple pills into bits a twentieth of a mg in size just to get by.

Occasionally one of the highly sophisticated radiation machines would fall out of calibration and shut itself down. When this happened there were long delays for patients receiving treatments from that machine while engineers worked to bring it back online. When a group of nurses and assistants appeared in the waiting area everyone knew one of the machines was out of order. We cringed in our chairs hoping it wasn't us they approached with a sorry expression and to politely inform us the delay of unknown length was ours to endure. This occurred three times out of my ten appointments. Twice it was my machine. The first time it happened there was a patient who made a big fuss. He insisted on skipping his treatment because it was Friday and he had a weekend getaway planned and with the delay would miss his flight. He was a man who did not accept his condition or simply didn't like being inconvenienced. He lashed out angrily at the nurse who was trying to console and persuade him to stay. She said his treatment was important and it wasn't a good idea to skip it. He left anyway. A few days later there was a second long delay. Jen and I passed the time talking with a couple from rural Washington. He was there to get radiation for bladder cancer for a second time around. She was his caretaker and memory bank as he was tired and forgetful. They spoke of their little retirement community situated at the end of a road where deer wander through yards and coyotes howl in the evening. They used golf carts to get around the neighborhood. Everyone knew everyone else. They had worked their entire lives for this little piece of paradise. Now they were staying in their grand-daughter's bedroom in a suburb south of Seattle and feeling guilty about inconveniencing her. But the writing was on the wall and they knew they wouldn't be returning home. They would have to put the house up for sale and move closer to town due to the advanced stage of his cancer. Their stories rang with sadness and melancholy. Though at one point she threw up her arms and said hopefully, "Who knows? Miracles happen every day." I hope they got the miracle they were looking for.

****

With cancer we are so suddenly thrown into a new reality it can be overwhelming. It can be difficult coming to grips with such an extreme situation. Getting a second or third opinion is a good idea if only to give oneself time to confirm but also to acclimate to this new reality. Had I any misgivings about my doctors and if things I was being told didn't jibe I would have sought a second or third opinion. Multiple myeloma is a rare cancer. It occurs randomly with no known cause. I couldn't have been luckier to be living in the same area of the country as one of the leading institutions for treating this cancer. It was obvious that they knew what they were doing. I was benefiting from the thousands of patients who came before me, and decades of research and experience on a disease that is a moving target.

We may see ourselves as victims at times but everything that happens in life requires a response. When bad things happen to us the quality of our response is vital. We choose how to respond and in our response we shrink or grow. Having to wait around for our treatments can be frustrating. It's unpleasant and one can feel like a cog in a machine. But as patients patience is what we need. We are on a schedule that is not of our own making and the only thing we control is how we react. I felt lucky to have Love Trust Gratitude Healing come to me in my moment of need. Something to focus on when the path was difficult and it was easy to waver when a situation was getting the best of me.

The old adage "without your health you have nothing" proves itself in spades when you get cancer. It is also true, unless you're alone, that your family is disrupted and they suffer along with you. Being on the cancer side of the equation I genuinely felt it was easier for me than for them. I was certainly thankful that it was me and not one of them. I prefer the active role. I can be a ham and the one with cancer is really an attention hog role. The way my family and friends beamed all that love at me, yes, I'll have some more of that.

****

"You are going to fight this?" "You're a warrior, you can beat it." "It's going to be a battle but you'll come out the victor." I don't how many times someone has tried to encourage me with some version of the above statements. As well, when someone famous dies of cancer the media is sure to convey that after facing their illness head-on and fighting fearlessly they lost their battle with cancer.

On the surface it sounds heroic to cast us as warriors, but describing our struggle with cancer (and many other challenges we face in life) as a fight, a battle, a war, doesn't give much insight into the experience and leaves only two possible outcomes: victory or defeat. What does this reveal of the person's encounter? Over the course of their illness they may have reached levels of love and redemption they never had before. Maybe it was the first time they realized the preciousness of their loved ones and they were able to communicate it to them. To experience their family and friends rally around them, offering whatever they could. They may have found peace and contentment before they passed, something they had never had in their lives. They wouldn't have had the opportunity had they died suddenly from a car accident, heart attack or the like. To me these are worse ways to die. They often leave vital things unsaid.

To be in a battle is to be in a state of tension and I believe this tension can be a barrier for healing. In my opinion remaining calm and relaxed should be the goal. Of course this isn't easy given the dire consequences we may be facing. But it does us good to let our medical team take care of the cancer while we love, laugh, dance, sing, eat and drink well.

Yes, cancer is a confrontation that demands an answer but it isn't to declare war. The experience is more akin to a surrender as we are carried along through the process as if on a conveyer belt while samples are taken, medicines injected, swallowed, infused, ports are spliced into us, and we are radiation beamed and chemo-dosed. For me a better response is love. We will probably never say we love our cancer, I certainly haven't, but we can appreciate the obstacle, the feeling that we have never wanted to live more, to say exactly how we feel to our family and friends, to marvel at how strong we are, surprisingly strong, incredibly strong. Even if we die it won't be because it got the better of us. We got the better of it. Can we love with all our might through this? Love is the only unlimited resource in the universe. We can fling it around willy nilly and our pockets will always be full. It is time to change the metaphor for cancer from war to something like dancing or singing. I used dance to replace war as the metaphor for my encounter with cancer. I'm not sure why I chose dance since I couldn't even walk maybe I chose it precisely for that reason. It didn't matter I only knew that I didn't want to use fight, battle or war to describe my experience. We must ask ourselves as a society; do we have to declare war on everything we don't like? Regarding cancer it won't make it any less dramatic, urgent or important, but it deserves more respect and its victims more than participants who can only win or lose.

****

I finished the last radiation treatment with no side effects other than fatigue. Indeed, fatigue was my constant companion throughout my experience. With the tumor gone there was no noticeable improvement in my numbness, balance or coordination. The damage was done. It had been a quick fall but looked to be a slow rise. A big question mark was how much of my former ability I would get back, assuming everything else went well and I lived long enough. I had to concentrate on every step I took, even with a cane and a wall or Jen's hand to steady me I could only go a short distance at a time. Still, I was happy to be alive and moving. I imagined having to use a cane the rest of my life and decided it would be okay. I might develop a suave and charming personality to go along with it. I imagined myself in a suit, wearing a fedora, and moving at an eighth of the speed of regular folks down a sidewalk in my head, saying, "Pardon me." "Oh, no, no, I'm fine, you go on ahead."

The second week in May I was at SCCA preparing for the first cycle of chemo that was to begin on the upcoming Friday. SCCA is located along the I-5 corridor on the north-end of downtown Seattle. The building is seven stories tall with a concave design facing north to take advantage of the view of Lake Union where sailboats angle back and forth across the water and seaplanes take off and land at regular intervals. When fog rolls in over the lake it is especially compelling. The waiting areas for the patients are laid out to take advantage of the view with floor-to-ceiling windows. This was indicative of what I saw as a patient-centric disposition.

My sister Patrice went out of her way to visit after hearing I had cancer. She flew in from Shanghai, China where she taught English at an international school. She came along with us to my appointments and helped Jen (who was doing everything at this point) as did our daughter, Ocean, who arrived a couple days later. Ocean kept the mood light and positive. It was good having some distraction leading into my first round of chemo but especially good for Jen who hadn't had a break in nearly a month.

Before the first cycle of chemo I had a CT scan (similar to an MRI except the tube is larger and it is much quieter), and a bone marrow aspiration to determine the percentage of multiple myeloma in my marrow. The aspiration involved a long needle poked through the hipbone into the marrow for extraction. The idea of long needles poking through flesh and bone is a stress-inducing prospect and with tension everything hurts more. During the procedure I focused on breathing deep and repeating my mantra. The specialist did a good job numbing the area but it stung and the sound of crunching bone wasn't pleasant either but it was better than I had imagined.

The idea of something unpleasant is usually worse than the reality. It's easy to understand that time spent in a fear-laden speculative mind is a waste, but staying out of it is incredibly difficult. I found myself tangled up in it all the time. When I was tired of repeating my mantra I would picture myself dancing. A salsa or a waltz usually came to mind though occasionally I would leap about like Baryshnikov. To be clear I was never much of a dancer, but in my head I could really go. I found it was useful to have a few ways to shift my attention when my mind ran amuck.

My chemo routine was a cocktail consisting of three different medicines taken over a twenty-eight day cycle. There was a daily pill called revlimid taken for the first twenty-one of the twenty-eight days. Every seven days I would receive an injection of bortezomib in the belly and a 40 mg dose of dexamethasone (yes, it was back but only one day a week). After twenty-eight days I would have one week off to recuperate while they determined the amount of multiple myeloma in my blood in order to measure the effectiveness of the medicines before starting the next cycle. A typical patient receives at least four to five cycles of chemo to reduce the percentage of multiple myeloma in the blood before moving on to the bone marrow transplant.

The morning of Friday, May 11, I took the first dose of dexamethasone at home and later in the day Jen drove us to SCCA to get my first shot of bortezomib. Before going to bed that night I swallowed the 25 mg revlimid pill. I knew what to expect from the dexamethasone though not in combination with the other medicines. Despite being fatigued and exhausted overall I figured it would still be difficult to sleep that night and I was right. I laid in bed while my mind ran laps around the room. At midnight I struggled out of bed, made my way to the living room, sat down with my laptop and started writing about this new reality with cancer. I wrote about my sudden loss of strength and mobility and the uncertainty the future held, but also the expanded perspective. I questioned how much pain would be involved going forward. Will the drugs cure me or kill me? That's what they were doing, killing healthy cells as well as cancer cells. And finally how in the world did I get this cancer? Was it due to the stress of the previous year when I was suffering from chronic elbow pain that limited my ability to write and virtually eliminated my ability to play the guitar? After raising the kids I was expecting to get out and play shows and see where it took me but it seemed my playing days were behind me. What was I going to do? A mid-fifties artist with few practical skills in a shrinking job market. I kicked myself for not picking up a trade or something in my youth that I could count on later. I certainly questioned all the decisions that had brought me to a dead end where everything fell apart because of a weak elbow. Was my immunity compromised during that angst period thus inducing my cancer? It didn't matter I suppose—a new reality was upon me. The direction of my life had altered so significantly. The length had as well. Those stresses from the year before seemed so distant and unimportant now. It was yet another lesson that worry is not only futile but also a waste of time and energy. While I was worrying about one thing something else was coming along.

Saturday morning found me as awake as the night before. The day passed with a slight buzz in my head from lack of sleep. That night I was up until dawn, again doing much the same as the night before. By Sunday the effects of the dexamethasone wore off and I slept the entire night. I woke Monday morning feeling physically and mentally exhausted with an acute sensitivity to light and sound. I knew that the range of responses to chemo are so varied that there was no way to know in advance exactly how my body would react. A major adjustment we have to make as cancer patients is the lack of certainty from our doctors regarding how treatments will affect us. We live in a society that expects easy answers and we are ripe for con artists who give them. Politicians come immediately to mind. But I've found throughout my life that there are no easy answers.

Every new physical sensation I felt put me on edge with the anticipation that it was going to get worse. Would I be one of the unlucky ones where the medicines cause so many bad symptoms I wouldn't be able to take them? Once again, I was caught up in fear and my symptoms grew worse, my light and sound sensitivity became unbearable, and suddenly my fingers were tingling and numb. Trapped in this fear, just repeating Love Trust Gratitude Healing wasn't effective in keeping me calm and centered. I began to explore each word pausing to list those I loved. I usually began with myself and moved outward: I love myself (It took me awhile to get used to saying I loved myself. It felt odd. I don't remember ever saying it before other than in jest), I love my family (saying each name), and my friends (again saying each name). I included neighbors, community, city, state, country, everyone on the planet including my enemies. I did the same with Trust: I trust myself to know I'm getting the right treatment. I trust my family and friends. I trust my medical team… And Gratitude: I'm grateful for my life, the lives of my family and friends… And Healing: I'm in need of healing, everyone is in need of some form of healing, the planet itself is in need of healing. I found this new exercise of LTGH helped me relax and with that my symptoms improved. By Tuesday I was feeling better except for the ever-present fatigue. Wednesday was better still and by Thursday I was feeling somewhat normal. On Friday the whole thing started again. Through all my rounds of chemo (there were four in all) I was on this weekly rollercoaster of energy.

****

I'm certain that staying calm and relaxed overall helped my body deal with the harsh treatments I was receiving and avoid so many of the more unpleasant side effects. My strength was focused on healing. I hadn't gotten any of the expected throat issues from the radiation and other than constipation (probably the worst part overall) and sound sensitivity during the first week of chemo I did well thereafter. Maybe I was lucky, I don't know, but I do know that having Love Trust Gratitude Healing to focus on instead of the woe of my situation gave me distance and perspective in dealing with the day-to-day.

There was an emphasis on staying active and hydrated during chemo. The hydration part was easy but the active part was difficult given my limited mobility. Despite this, every few hours I grabbed my cane, hobbled over to the nearest wall, and moved from the living room through the dining room into the kitchen and back again. Forty-nine steps equaled one lap. Fifty laps equalled about a mile. I was nowhere near doing that many laps but that was my goal. It was tedious but I was moving and there was much to be satisfied with that.

I tracked the days and weeks of the chemo round. With each passing week I was another twenty-five percent of the way through. I counted down the twenty-one revlimid pills in the bottle, looking forward to no pills after the third week. I would be seventy-five percent of the way through the round. It felt good knowing the fourth and final week entailed only the dexamethasone and bortezomib injection. I must admit I have a strong aversion to taking pills so the idea of taking a chemo pill was a challenge. That's why I waited until it was time for bed and I had no choice. I swallowed it with a large glass of water, then drank another, thinking my body could use the extra hydration.

After I was diagnosed and started the rapid schedule of treatments I kept my attention on what was right in front of me. I seldom looked ahead. I was aware of the bone marrow transplant but hadn't looked into what it entailed. For the longest time I took it literally, wondering how they would get all the bone marrow out of my bones and how would they fill them back up. I pictured a long piece of metal with a spoon on the end scraping out the old marrow and another long piece of metal with a blunt end stuffing in the new. It was unsettling to think about. In any case when I finished the first round of chemo I had it in my head that was that and we would be moving on to the transplant. But when we met with Dr. Cowan and discovered another round of chemo was pending I realized this would go on for a while. When I asked how long, he said he didn't know. It depended on the measure of multiple myeloma in the bloodstream known as its M-spike. Once again I was reminded that there are no solid answers when it comes to cancer treatments.

The second round of chemo was better than the first. That isn't to say it was great but at least I had a plan in place to deal with the constipation and I was familiar with how my body reacted to the weekly drug regimen. I rode the wave of energy and fatigue. My sleepless Friday and Saturday nights were devoted to all-night writing and music sessions. Sunday night through Tuesday I caught up on my sleep. I started having lucid dreams of walking again. I dreamt of ambling up the side of a steep hill or across a field, feeling so elated and thinking I shouldn't be able to do this but I am. I woke up wondering if my dreams were taunting me. The hopeful side of me thought maybe my subconscious mind knew something. I'm convinced that this was the case. In fact I believe my unconscious mind was aware of my cancer long before it manifested as a tumor and came to my conscious attention. My evidence is the songs I was writing six months earlier one of which was titled *Draw Blood*. The album I imagined at the time though never finished was to have the same name with a streak of my blood across the cover. I don't think it was a coincidence but my unconscious expressing that something wasn't right with my blood. Maybe I will amble down a hill again in this lifetime or at least be able to walk up the street on my own. That would be so amazing. I've been such an antsy, active person my entire life. I've always had a tough time keeping still. It would be incredible to move again unencumbered. But for now I had no alternative but to learn stillness.

****

Through the cycles of chemo I spent most of the time lying in bed watching television (I burned through hours of Netflix), reading, or just thinking. I realized that the healing I was experiencing was less physical and more emotional and spiritual. The last of the reservoir of anger I inherited from my dad had dissipated. The conclusion I reached during this period was that even though we may be breaking down physically we can continue to grow spiritually and emotionally and express it all the way to the end of our lives.

With time all things disintegrate on the physical level. Cancer can be an accelerated form of that process. Time is always running out. Treating the physical body may add to that time but what then? It is still winding down and this is true for everyone. Cancer takes what for us is an ambiguous thing and makes it definitive. Our mortality appears before us as if to say, "Here I am as always, now what?" Like I've said, everyone is in need of some form of healing. It can be emotional, spiritual or physical. It makes sense to me to expand the focus from just healing the body, which can go either way, to healing emotionally and spiritually as well which I think is the most effective use of Love Trust Gratitude Healing. The two graphs on the next page illustrate this point.

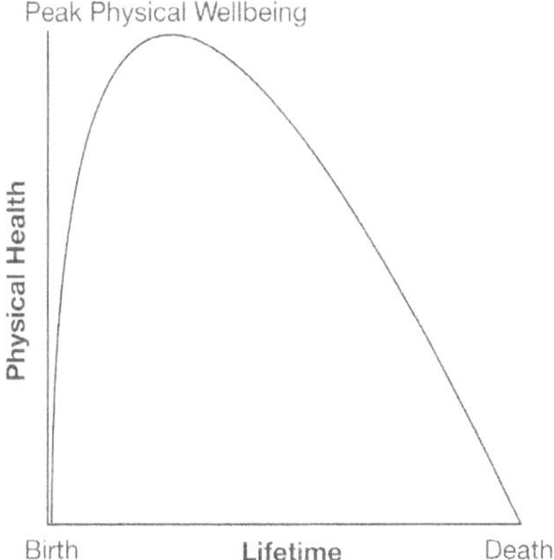

The above graph illustrates the typical journey our physical body takes over a lifetime. Hopefully we enjoy at or near peak health for as long as possible but inevitably our bodies breakdown over time.

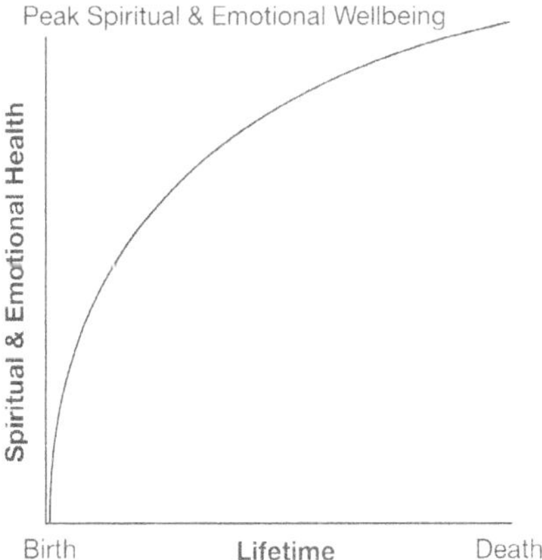

The above graph illustrates the potential of our spiritual and emotional healing all the way to our death. Even though our physical bodies breakdown our spiritual and emotional healing can continue and even accelerate. As well, this healing can be passed on to our loved ones and so on. Healing that continues long after we are gone.

I now believe that spiritual and emotional healing can occur right to the end of our lives and continue on through our loved ones after we pass. This is something my dad failed to do in his lifetime. Even when he had the chance on his deathbed he denied himself and me intimacy and healing by lying in an attempt to save face. A face that would soon be gone. A history of pain and suffering in a family can turn on a word or meaningful gesture. It can be as simple as saying, "I'm sorry." My dad couldn't or wouldn't do that. His life remained unresolved emotionally and spiritually. It's his great tragedy but affected me as well.

****

In July after the second round of chemo Dr. Cowan informed us everything was moving in the right direction. My blood work was looking good. I was no longer anemic. Other than the usual fatigue I was feeling pretty good. I was able to walk short distances without a cane with the exception of stairs and uneven surfaces. I didn't stray far from a wall or object I could reach for when I began to lose my balance. It still took a concerted effort to take each step but I was improving. I started physical therapy hoping to accelerate my progress. My wildest dream was to walk normally again. That would be a huge prize. It's an interesting experience to fall so low that returning to my former regular old self seemed like such a massive gift. There has to be a country song out there called *You don't know what you got till its gone* or *Just gimme back what I had Lord and I'll be fine.*

My physical therapist gave me routines for reengaging my dormant back muscles and various balancing exercises that included standing on one leg or in tandem (one foot in front of the other) and sidestepping with a resistance band around my ankles. Balancing for more than a few seconds was extraordinarily difficult. For safety she recommended that I do my balance routines next to the kitchen counter so I could catch myself before I tumbled over. It still boggled my mind that something so easy my entire life was now so frustratingly difficult.

I had the double task of dealing with cancer and learning to walk again, but walking gave me an immediate thing to concentrate on other than my cancer. My general antsy-ness paid dividends in my recovery as it forced me out of bed more often to walk my laps helping my balance and coordination improve as well as benefiting my physical recovery from the cancer and its treatments. In little chunks over the course of a day I was walking at least a mile inside the house.

****

I received good news after the third round of chemo. The numbers showed there was barely a presence of multiple myeloma in my blood—less than 0.2 percent M-spike. I figured at this point we would go forward with the bone marrow transplant, but after some discussion and the fact that my body was reacting so positively to the treatments it was recommended that I go one more round to see if it could be reduced further still. I was disappointed. I had it in mind that I would be starting the bone marrow transplant in late summer when the weather was good rather than fall, when the weather turned rainy and flu season began. A fourth round of chemo would take me through the end of August into September. With a month to prep, the transplant wouldn't happen until mid October. I would have to carry through the fall and winter months with little or no immunity.

Since my diagnosis I had received good news through all my treatments. The tumor was gone. I was no longer anemic. Despite the chemo my blood work was normal. Multiple myeloma cells were barely detectable in my blood. I was walking without a cane. In the past when it came to good news I had the tendency to think, this can't last, it's sure to even out. I never think that when bad news comes knocking. In that case I'm inclined to think it will go on forever. Now I think I was taking personal the up down wave-like nature of life. Will this wave crash on the beach sooner or later? Who knows? But everything pointed to a long ride so until I heard further or suddenly felt worse I would continue to expect good news through the fourth round and beyond the bone marrow transplant.

The fourth round of chemo went like the previous two. It had become routine. I walked, did my physical therapy routine (I was now doing the Electric Slide to improve coordination—I was dancing!). I wrote, played guitar and sang. Summer waned. Fall was coming and so was the bone marrow transplant.

After the fourth round of chemo Jen and I met with Dr. Cowan. He gave us the fantastic news that there was no measurable multiple myeloma in my blood. Technically I was in remission. Only about ten percent of patients hit remission before their bone marrow transplant. Again, I credit the ability to stay calm and relaxed overall thanks to my family, my meditation on Love Trust Gratitude Healing, and of course my medical team—the treatments they provided were the direct confrontation with the cancer inside my body. By staying well fed, hydrated, calm and active I maintained an environment with the potential for the best healing.

****

As I've said before, cancer strips you down to your core being and magnifies the essentials in your life. Those essentials are not many compared to the laundry list we carry around most of our lives. Those essentials for me are: family, friends, good food, shelter, meaningful work, the sun, the moon, Love Trust Gratitude Healing.

From diagnosis onward I experienced a period of heightened aliveness with bouts of elation. The world stuck out in sharp relief. I was in awe of the simplest things. The wind moving through the trees, leaves dancing in response. Watching a pair of pileated woodpeckers flying through the foliage, stopping here and there, tapping sections of bark before moving on brought me to tears. From my wheelchair rolling down the hospital corridors or on the elevator I had been compelled to meet everyone's eyes with my own in order to communicate that I saw them and was happy to see them, "We're alive isn't it great!" I had an overwhelming love for everyone and everything. I still do, but the almost evangelical intensity I felt at the time has faded. This period lasted through the end of radiation and into my fourth round of chemo when one day I found myself getting upset as I was struggling through my physical therapy routine. Progress had stalled despite my effort. I was told the largest gains are made in the first year after spinal compression. The year was ticking away and I still couldn't balance on one leg for more than a few seconds. I could walk without a cane for only short distances at a time but it still required the utmost concentration with eyes looking straight ahead or down at my feet. If I turned my head to either side I immediately lost my balance. I caught hold of myself when I realized it was the first time I had felt negative since my diagnosis and that just a couple months before when I was still getting around with a cane I was grateful for that. But there I was whining about the slow progress despite the fact that I was making progress. This confrontation with cancer is an up and down affair. Frustration and fear comes and goes even with a mantra. I was caught up in my expectations yet again and impatient for results. We humans are dynamic self-reflecting beings. It isn't easy being us. We get bound up in the past or future, forgetting the present where all life/action occurs. After catching myself in the act of desiring what I didn't have right then and there I laughed. I hadn't expected to remain at such a lofty height of openness and love forever. My life had fifty-some-odd-years of trajectory to account for. As I became acclimated to my cancer and treatments I was naturally falling back into my regular old self, wiser perhaps, but still Mr. Antsy Pants.

Every life has momentum and even getting cancer doesn't alter the path for some. I remember a patient in the waiting area of Radiation Oncology. A woman in her forties accompanied by another woman around the same age who may have been her sister—they looked alike. She was wearing cut-off jean shorts and a large Seahawks football jersey. Her legs were covered with scabs and bruises. She kept jumping out of her chair and disappearing into the hallway through the sliding glass doors for varying lengths of time before returning to her seat. Her sister tailed behind at some distance out the door and back again. After a third round trip she began digging through her purse. Not finding what she was looking for she dropped her purse on the floor, stood, rifled through the pockets of her cutoffs then turned toward her seat and searched the cushions of her chair. She returned to her purse for another frantic search and still not finding what she was looking for she got up and left with her sister following close behind pleading for her to stay. It was obvious that she was an addict of some kind and my heart went out to her. The momentum of her addiction was overwhelming her reality and ability to deal with whatever health issues were present.

I've always liked a challenge more than an easy chair and I suspect that's true for many others. There is something wonderful about being deeply engaged in an activity where the outcome is uncertain. Well, I sure found the ultimate challenge of uncertainty by getting cancer and losing the ability to walk. It was life or death. The highest hurdle. As I said earlier when I made the decision that I chose my parents, a great burden lifted as most of my childhood resentments were transformed. But can I say that I chose this cancer? I don't think I can even though I recognize that it would be the more powerful position.

I was able to laugh at my frustration over the slow progress of walking again and recognize that though frustration and uncertainty are part of life I could still be curious and open and let it go. Through the rounds of chemo my love had deepened. I was solid in my trust. I was so grateful for everyone in my life. My perspective had broadened and I was healing emotionally, spiritually and physically. I was lucky. These were all positives that I was gaining from my confrontation with cancer. If I died in the short term I wouldn't say that it was a loss when I've gained so much. I wanted to communicate it to my family and friends and anyone who would listen. I was more convinced than ever that the answer to the fundamental confrontations in life is not to battle but to dance. By dance I mean life for life's sake or movement without agenda. Like some forms of martial arts where one doesn't confront an opponent head-on but uses their energy and momentum against them.

****

The bone marrow transplant process started almost immediately after my fourth round of chemo. The radiation treatments and then chemo were the main reasons I hadn't made much progress walking. The fact that I would be weakened further still by the high dose chemo called mephalan involved with the transplant meant the aspect of improving my walking was practically nil. I hoped given my remission status that they would take me aside and tell me the bone marrow transplant was unnecessary so I could get on with the difficult work of regaining my balance and coordination. That wasn't the case though of course I could choose not to do it and apparently there are other cancer institutes that were opting to forgo bone marrow transplants for multiple myeloma patients in favor of just putting them on some type of a low dose chemo maintenance program. I asked Dr. Cowan if he were in my shoes would he go through with the transplant and without hesitation he said he would. I knew I should go through with it myself as it was still the best chance of surviving this dreadful disease long term. My trust in Dr. Cowan and the incredible people at SCCA had gotten me this far in good stead, I was going the whole way through.

For the bone marrow transplant I was transferred to the sixth floor of SCCA. My transplant would be handled by a medical staff associated with Fred Hutchinson Cancer Research. Here again I was lucky just by living in Seattle because Fred Hutch is one of the pioneering institutes for bone marrow transplants. As well, I would be home in my own bed during the process unlike so many who travel to Seattle for treatment and stay at a residential hotel or the like.

Bone marrow transplants are a serious life-and-death business and I felt that when I arrived on the sixth floor. It had a more somber vibe overall. I was assigned to the Aqua team led by Dr. Holmberg. She missed our first meeting because of a cold. Any ailment, even a mild cold kept members of the staff away from the sixth floor because there were patients at various stages of their transplants who were severely immunosuppressed and vulnerable to even the smallest infection or virus. Jen and I met with Dr. Holmberg's associate Dr. Appelbaum and Aqua team nurse Jennifer. We were given binders of information regarding the transplant process as well as consent forms. Dr. Appelbaum was friendly and naturally inquisitive, asking questions about my life including being a musician. Then he gave a brief history on the development of bone marrow transplants and the difficulties overcome. In the beginning one had about a fifty-fifty chance of survival. Now patient's chances were well over ninety percent. There would be tests measuring organ function to see if I was a good candidate for the transplant. Dr. Appelbaum had been working at Fred Hutch since the mid-seventies. He was there when multiple myeloma was an apex killer and through all the advances and breakthroughs in treatments for this deadly disease. He spoke of promising new medical treatments on the horizon. I must admit most of what he told me went right over my head. In these matters it often comes down to do I trust that they know what they're doing and it was obvious to me they did.

Through mid September and into October I underwent a litany of tests (heart, lungs, liver, kidney, teeth) to determine my viability for undergoing the transplant. Once the green light was given there were classes on hygiene, nutrition, and food preparation. I was told what to expect as well as symptoms to look out for in the early days post transplant. There was a list of emergency phone numbers, day numbers, after-hours numbers, in case something went awry. An absolute necessity was a full time caretaker as I would be considerably weakened by the high dose chemo. I needed another pair of eyes to see and hands to help because there was no telling what might happen post transplant. Jen had been my caretaker up to this point and there was no way she was giving the job away to someone else, even when I suggested it might be too much to handle.

I was relieved to discover the bone marrow transplant didn't involve scraping out the old marrow and stuffing in the new. I'm not sure if the actual procedure was any better. The one I would undergo was called autologous (ah tah luh jus). This transplant involved collecting my stem cells from my bloodstream, after they are forced out of the bone marrow where they normally reside. They are then cryogenically frozen for preservation. When the time was right, usually within a few weeks, I would receive a dose of mephalan that would wipe out the multiple myeloma along with my bone marrow and its capacity to regrow cells. To do all this high volume blood work a catheter (called a Hickman line for the man who invented it; Dr. Robert Hickman) had to be grafted to a large vein in my chest. Jen and I spent a Saturday morning at UW Medical for this minor surgical procedure. After checking in at the front desk we were led to a curtained medical bay with a gurney bed. After putting on a hospital gown and crawling into bed I was prepped, then wheeled to surgery. They shaved and scrubbed an area up near my collar bone on the right side of my chest. Local anesthesia was applied where the vein they were after was located and the Hickman was spliced in, stitched in place, and covered with a square of see-through plastic dressing. The dressing would need to be changed weekly. My skin reddened underneath the plastic and itched most of the time. The Hickman had a line in and a line out and once in place all my blood draws were taken through it. Blood vials filled in an instant. We were told it wouldn't be good if a line were to split open or a valve became contaminated. Therefore extra instruction went into showing us how to care for it. This involved cleaning the valves and flushing the lines daily—chores that fell to Jen. I held the lines and operated the on/off switches, gave encouragement, and watched while she cleaned the tip of each valve with an alcohol swab then attached a syringe of saline solution and flushed the line. I felt a cool sensation when the saline solution entered my bloodstream.

We face so many procedures during cancer treatments that seem difficult if not impossible to endure. I discovered again that the anticipation of these procedures was worse than the reality. When they have to fire a beam of radiation at your tumor, poke a needle through your hip bone for some marrow, or splice a two way catheter in your chest, you can get caught up in a web of fear and anxiety. Again I found that the idea of having the Hickman grafted to my chest was worse than the reality. It wasn't pleasant but I endured it and there were times when I forgot it was there.

Many patients come to name the extraneous parts that are attached to their person. It's a good practice and way to find humor or personalization in procedures that are physically invasive. I considered naming my Hickman Porter Waggoner after the old country music star. One can face and get through a lot of seemingly impossible obstacles with calmness, acceptance and a good sense of humor.

****

It's the children with cancer who go through their ordeal with the most nobility, honesty and openness. I got the chance to observe them in the waiting area on the sixth floor. These amazing kids displayed a dignity and grace that put to shame more than a few of the adult cancer patients who clearly showed they were suffering over their suffering. As adults we drag around decades of life. All our triumphs and failures and resentments and shoulda beens and coulda beens and mighta beens and now this had to happen. The children on the other hand just wanted to play and they did despite being hampered by their little catheters, ports and fatigue. A little girl around two or three years old would stand in front of her mom's chair and dance waving her arms over her head and bouncing on her feet. She confirmed for me my choice of dancing in response to what ailed me.

The parents of the children carried themselves remarkably well through what could only be profound unrelenting stress and anxiety. Observing these incredible families led me to realize that a meaningful life is not measured in years. Like a mayfly, some of these children will blink in and out of the world but that makes them shine all the brighter. The impact and meaning of their brief time here may be all the more profound and impactful on the lives of their parents, brothers, sisters, doctors and nurses, everyone who crosses their path. This was further confirmed for me by a nurse I met post transplant who described an experience she had with a remarkable boy of twelve she cared for thirty years previously. She spoke of his situation, his openness and honesty as he faced certain death. "He would have been forty-two this year," she said with tears in her eyes, "I'll never forget him." Truly the children impacted the older patients waiting for their appointments. I know they impacted me and I'm the better for it. They have my deepest love, respect, and appreciation for their lives. My heart goes out to all who have suffered this fate. Cancer taking a loved one early does not in any way diminish the meaning of their life. More time does not equal more meaningfulness. That's why kids play and we should as well, no matter the circumstances.

The children give us good reason for not putting off until later what we should be doing right now. Cancer brings us face to face with our lives. It makes clear what has always been true, we are going to pass out of this world someday and not by our own discretion. It's easy to push this condition of life aside, leave things for another day, because we may have a high probability of getting through our twenties, thirties, forties, even our fifties and sixties. We can go for years drifting along through routine and habit only to get cancer or something else and discover what is of ultimate importance to us. I can guarantee it isn't routine and habit. There is never a good reason to put off making a life instead of just making a living. It's always time for love, dance, to do what must be done and say what must be said.

****

In the weeks leading up to my transplant Jen and I were at SCCA or UW hospital nearly every day, and sometimes twice a day if there was an appointment in the morning at SCCA and another at UW hospital in the afternoon. I was beholden to a schedule that was relentless, knowing that after the transplant it would be more so. We would be at SCCA every day for blood draws and to check-in with Aqua team to see how everything was going.

Stem cells reside in our bone marrow where they produce various blood cells. In order to collect them they must be pushed out into the bloodstream. For this I was given a shot once a day for three days that promoted exponential growth of my stem cells, causing millions to spill out into my bloodstream. I was told that my bones would feel the pressure of that growth and it was true. They ached like crazy, reminiscent of the growing pains I experienced in my youth. After three days it was determined that there were enough stem cells in my blood to proceed with the collection and I was given consecutive morning appointments for what would be a slow eight to ten hour process over several days. The goal was to collect enough stem cells for two transplants. A bone marrow transplant requires a minimum of five million stem cells.

The morning of my first appointment Jen and I arrived with books to read in expectation of a long day. We were escorted to a medical bay the size of a large cubicle that contained a sink, a medical supply cabinet, the stem cell extraction machine, a tv hanging high up in the corner, a bed for me and a chair for Jen. Both lines of my Hickman were attached to the machine and I laid in the bed while it cycled through my blood, extracted my stem cells depositing them in a plastic pouch that hung on a hook. It was noisy affair that made reading difficult so we opted for a selection of DVDs they had on hand and whiled away our time watching several of *The Borne Identity* series. The noise of the machine drowned out most of the dialog though it wasn't difficult to follow as it was mostly action and the good and bad guys were clearly demarcated. Yet again I was lucky because after only one session of six hours they had gathered enough for two transplants. They collected 11.6 million stem cells during that one session.

I found out the next day that the following week, Wednesday, October 17, I would receive the mephalan through my Hickman line. I had the usual jump in nervous energy with this most dramatic and intense procedure pending. The idea of it is extreme. You get what amounts to a lethal dose, a scorched earth technique, of chemo that would certainly kill you if you didn't have your harvested stem cells or they failed to engraph. It's a heady experience to face and easy to get stressed about. I knew my speculative mind would be working overtime conjuring up all sorts of awful possibilities. I meditated on LTGH, thought about the kids with cancer and the measure of a meaningful life, the positive results achieved with a high quality response, and just plain luck, luck I hoped would hold out as long as possible.

A major side effect of mephalan is mucositis, which is an inflammation of cells in the mouth, throat and gastrointestinal tract causing open sores, bleeding, thick salvia, and making it difficult to swallow. Over time it was discovered that holding ice chips in the mouth prior to, during, and after chemo often reduced its severity by constricting the blood flow and limiting the amount of chemo to that area. I took it to heart and although they recommended it be done for five to six hours I ice-chipped for eleven hours that day. Forty-eight hours later, the time it took for the chemo to clear my system, half of my harvested stem cells were thawed and infused into my bloodstream through the Hickman line. There is a preservative added to the stem cells prior to freezing that emits the smell of garlic or canned corn through the skin for days after the cells are back in the body. The odor is strong and a telltale sign for anyone working on the sixth floor that the person who just passed them in the hall has recently undergone a bone marrow transplant. I threw up after the last of my stem cells entered my bloodstream. I threw up several times a day for the next few weeks as the effects of the mephalan kicked in.

After the transplant it became a waiting game for the stem cells to settle back into my bones, reattach themselves and start producing new blood cells. This typically takes 14 to 21 days. During this phase I was at SCCA every day giving blood and meeting with my able and always professional Aqua team to see how I was doing. I could see by the numbers that my white cell blood count was going down daily. Soon it would be at or near zero. In the meantime I was highly susceptible to infection. Even a cold virus could be deadly. A fever was the number one thing we had to look out for. Anything above 100.9 degrees warranted a call to SCCA and a stay at UW hospital. The transplant itself can cause a spike in temperature just for its harsh impact on the body. We took my temperature three times a day. It fluctuated between my normal temperature of 97.6 and 99.9 degrees. Extreme fatigue had set in by this point and it was a miserable waiting game. Time crawled. There was really nothing I could do but struggle to eat, drink, sleep, and stay calm and relaxed which was not easy given the precarious situation. As the days wore on my temperature flirted with 100 degrees then seven days after the transplant I pegged a temperature of 101 degrees and was on my way to UW hospital. A large percentage of patients end up in the hospital for at least a few days given the severity of bone marrow transplants.

We were told to bypass the emergency room and go straight to the seventh floor cancer ward where they would be expecting me. It was early Saturday evening and the UW Huskies football team were playing in their stadium next door. The traffic was terrible and delayed us getting to the hospital. I sat in the passenger seat with my eyes closed, breathing deep and trying to relax. We inched along Jen scanning ahead for parking. Every parking lot was full. Jen dropped me at the entrance and went off in search of parking. I was back where I started this journey seven months ago. This time I walked in under my own power.

On the seventh floor I was given a room and an IV was attached to the Hickman line for the rest of my stay. My hair began to fall out in bunches. It was all over my pillow and half of it seemed to find its way into my mouth. One of the nurses was kind enough to buzzcut the rest of it. Soon even that stubble was gone. Yet again it was no time for vanity.

I wasn't happy to be back in the hospital just because of those dreaded hospital beds. I had hoped I could ride it out at home in my own bed. A couple days later when mucositis developed in the back of my throat and my white blood cell count hit zero I was glad to be there. Three days in particular were especially harsh as fatigue like I had never experienced before took hold and swallowing was damn near impossible. A morphine hookup was attached to my IV stand and I was given a button to push when symptoms became intolerable. The morphine dose was tightly regulated by quantity and a timer that released the drug over intervals of fifteen or twenty minutes. I had some interesting dreams.

Yet again I found with this experience when it comes to pain and discomfort the way through is surrender. It boils down to acceptance. It releases tension caused by the pain. This is where I am and this is how it feels. To relax when confronted by pain is difficult. I was constipated from all the meds, achy from head to toe, always throwing up, enduring the mucositis. Repeating Love Trust Gratitude Healing I found a third exercise. When listing those that I loved I began listing what I loved about them. I did the same with trust and gratitude. It kept me out of the weeds of fearful speculation most of the time. Also, despite the enormous fatigue, at least twice a day, I forced myself to get up and walk the halls, pushing or pulling my IV contraption on wheels along with me.

Jen was with me every day in my hospital room, coming in the morning and leaving in the early evening. She made the days tolerable just being there. Since it was around halloween we spent our time watching horror movies from the seventies and eighties on television. It was great fun and a useful distraction watching movies we hadn't seen since we were young. Most of them were pretty cheesy and we enjoyed moaning and groaning over the bad special effects and unconvincing and silly plot-lines.

The first line of defense against infection are cells in the bloodstream called neutrophils. These cells are short-lived, surviving from a few hours to a day or so. It was their numbers that were monitored closely. After they hit zero in my bloodstream we waited nervously for their numbers to rebound which they did after those three miserable days. It's difficult to convey the relief I felt when their numbers reappeared in my blood. They increased steadily afterward indicating that my stem cells had engraphed. I was exactly fourteen days post transplant. The most vulnerable time had passed. I marveled at my body's strength and endurance in handling everything that had been thrown at it the past seven months. Radiation, chemo, bone marrow transplant, one after the other with less than a week off in between. The intensity of it really hit me afterwards. During the entire process I continued to focus on what was right there in front of me. I left it to Dr. Cowan and then Dr. Holmberg to deal with the cancer while I took on the task of staying calm, relaxed and drinking in this beautiful gift called life. A couple days later I was back home, on the way to normal blood cell counts again.

The bone marrow transplant knocked out my immunity built up over the years. I had the immunity of a new born baby and was advised to eat only well cooked food and severely restrict my exposure to people in general and crowds in particular. For three months following the transplant I was on a immunosuppressed diet. I avoided eating out for food safety reasons and generally restricted myself to cooking at home. I consumed lots of protein to help my muscles, damaged by the chemo, recover their strength. Eating was not a pleasure but a chore. The transplant had wiped out my tastebuds (they returned about four months post transplant). Everything tasted dull and unappetizing.

The months following the transplant my fatigue was up and down. There were days when I felt almost normal. The muscle knots I had suffered from for so many months were gone. Except for my gimpy elbow I felt no pain. I was astonished I had made it this far in such a short time, though when I was in the middle of it it seemed to drag on forever. I know to some degree it will drag on for the rest of my life. This is the burden with incurable diseases but I hope if it comes again I can walk through it instead of crawling into it.

There was a drop-off in appointments beginning in December. I was still fragile but all the big hurdles were behind me. I had been so busy the previous nine months, with a packed schedule of appointments and treatments and measurements and blood draws that propelled me forward I had little time for anything else. In a way it had become my life. Not to mention the relationships I had built with the medical personnel, seeing them nearly every day. All of that dropped away so suddenly I was melancholy for a few weeks.

And more tired than I realized. Sleeping in and taking afternoon naps were the norm for a while.

A few months after the transplant hair like fine silk appeared on my scalp. As time went on it grew thicker, coarser and curly. I have a different head of hair. Maybe it's temporary but at least Jen likes it. The winter months in Seattle are cold and rainy which was something I had to avoid in my vulnerable state so I bought a cheap treadmill to help with my walking indoors where it was warm and dry. The treadmill provided a flat uniform surface to walk on and hand rails to steady myself while I practiced walking and turning my head at the same time. I walked every day and eventually I was able to turn my head from side to side without holding the rails or losing my balance. By March my balance and coordination had improved dramatically. Oh the gratitude I felt just to be able to walk again! Not as well as I used to but well enough to marvel about it. And almost every day since even when I'm simply walking to the kitchen, I smile and exclaim "I'm walking!" In a way I repeated the toddler experience of transitioning from crawling to the precarious act of walking. I felt again the triumph one sees in the eyes of a toddler when they take their first steps. What a gift it is to put one foot in front of the other and move. Where for so long I could only dance in my head now I could dance on my feet. Love Trust Gratitude Healing.

****

Looking back to the time before I collapsed to the floor I now realized I was having symptoms that indicated something was wrong, yet I never went to the doctor. I'm not saying a doctor would have dug deep enough to find my multiple myeloma based on telling them I had painful muscle knots but I'll never know now. Instead I searched the internet. My painful muscle knots corresponded with locations in the body called pressure points. Following this thread I watched chiropractor videos on youtube which led me to routines involving rolling over the pressure points with rubber balls among other exercises meant to release the knots. I did this for months, meanwhile the knots didn't improve. I reasoned that they occurred because of over-exercising or not stretching enough and that it would take a long time to heal since I was getting older and that goes with the territory yada yada yada. This is how searching the internet led me astray and delayed my seeking professional help. I came up with all kinds of reasons for my pain that were perfectly logical at the time. All of them were wrong. Had I been less sure of the stories I was telling myself maybe I would have sought other opinions, instead, it took me falling to the floor unable to walk to get me to a doctor. As I recall I was still in denial thinking it was a slipped disc that somehow I didn't feel. Surely I would know if I had slipped a disc, but again the stories I told myself. I know I'm not alone in this. Over 40 percent of folks who are told by a doctor that they have some form of cancer go into denial. This denial and the obvious delay in treatment it brings may prove catastrophic for them and their loved ones as it almost did for me. Even folks not in denial about their cancer, if they go looking on the internet, may come to believe that they can juice their cancer away, eat more veggies, or something like that. A nurse once told me of a woman in her thirties with two young children who was treating her breast cancer with yoga. I don't want to denigrate anyone's choice on how to deal with their cancer but when it comes to the physical nature of the human body western medicine has few rivals. I heard many different languages spoken in the waiting areas by folks from all over the world seeking treatment at SCCA.

****

The opposite of my experience with cancer was endured by one of my oldest and dearest friends, Hap Mansfield. As I was recovering from my bone marrow transplant she called with terrible news that she had massive blood clots in her lungs. One evening around Thanksgiving suddenly she couldn't breathe. She called 911 and was taken to emergency where they discovered the blood clots. She was put on blood thinners. They also found dark spots on her bladder and elsewhere in her body that they could do nothing about until the blood clots were dealt with. As was her nature she downplayed the seriousness of the situation but I knew her mom had passed from bladder cancer about fifteen years previously and that she was susceptible to the same. I feared that it had already metastasized or would before the blood clots cleared up.

I met Hap over the phone in the early nineties when I was in a band in Seattle and she was the editor of a small national music magazine published out of Minneapolis. She had given my band's first record a good review and I was calling to see if the magazine had received our follow up record. Hap answered the phone and let me tell you there was no one in the world like her. A more open, enthusiastic and curious person I've yet to meet. We struck up an instant friendship. A short while later we discovered we shared the same birthday, nine years apart. She was unique in the overwhelming generosity she offered everyone she came in contact with. In a world of mostly me-first people she was a you-first person. She was the type who took the smaller portion of food or ate the burnt piece of toast that no one else wanted. In her twenties she was diagnosed as bipolar but struggled under the yoke of medications. In her case, the negatives outweighed the positives including her opinion of her doctors. Eventually she stopped taking pills and turned to meditation, and to a large degree of success. We worked together on projects over the years. She helped edit my books and was a strong supporter of my more adventurous music. She became an important member of our family. Jen, Ocean and Bluewolf loved her dearly as well.

We spoke sporadically and only a few minutes at a time over the months because she was fatigued. She said it was because of the blood thinning medications but now I know it was also the bladder cancer which was moving along unabated. In February she called with good news that the blood clots were gone and they would now begin to deal with her bladder. In March, April, and May we spoke seldom as she was usually sapped from the treatments. Then in early June I got the horrible news that she was moving to hospice. The bladder cancer had metastasized. They didn't know how long she had. It could be a year. It could be a month. When Jen and I spoke with her in mid June her voice had weakened significantly. Her legs had weakened as well and now she was bedridden. We last spoke on our birthdays, June 24. She died less than two weeks later. Just like that she was whisked out of the world. It was heartbreaking. We miss her so much.

For each of us it makes a difference what type of cancer we have, the stage, support at home, financials, insurance. There are so many variables throwing obstacles in a difficult path. Still, there are gifts. As it takes away, it gives. Through our confrontation with cancer we find out who we really are and what we're made of. We get the chance to shed all the petty hangups and bullshit in our lives. And deeper still there's the expanded perspective. The realization that life and death are two parts of the same whole. That we don't know when our number will come up so we should act accordingly. We discover how strong we are in taking on radiation, chemo, surgeries, often at the same time. That a meaningful life can't be measured in years. To learn and appreciate the value of helplessness. To take this experience as an opportunity to heal emotionally and spiritually even if we can't physically. I have heard cancer survivors express that they had no desire to return to their pre-cancer selfs. Why is that? I can't speak for everyone but I believe it's the afore-mentioned gifts among others they discovered and carry with them from the experience. It is in line with that old saying what doesn't kill you makes you stronger. That's not to say they didn't have more than few dark moments after diagnosis and during treatments. All struggles are up and down. It means that the gifts brought by the struggle were life changing in positive ways. Folks who get the wake up call from cancer and survive are not likely to squander their second chance. All that said, I know there are cancer experiences that are so horrific little positivity is gained. Life isn't fair...

The optimal path is to let our medical team deal with the cancer. The way for us to confront our cancer is from the inside with the rich inner life we built over the years. Whether we know it or not it's there waiting to be tapped. It's there to confirm that we don't lose because we might not make it into our seventies, eighties or nineties.

I think that Jen as both my partner and caretaker carried the greater burden over the course of my illness. Especially because it began with my losing the ability to walk and suddenly she had to do everything. She also began using Love Trust Gratitude Healing as a mantra to take herself out of fearful speculation. There are perhaps a dozen or so other folks who are also using LTGH as a mantra (I was struck by how many people I told about Love Trust Gratitude Healing who responded so positively and seemed to recognize its usefulness). She handled it all magnificently but I suspect that as I get back to my normal self she's bound to have a letdown of some kind. It was traumatic for her having to see me fall so abruptly out of good health. And then watch as I went through procedure after procedure and struggled to regain my health, balance and coordination. She was there for it all much of the time feeling helpless. She also had to worry about an uncertain future and one possibly without me. Now that most of the initial journey is behind me it is important that I take care of her. I think it's the last step we have to take if our caretaker is a loved one. It will be nice to get the focus off of me. I've had enough of this attention-hog role I was dealt.

One or two years out from cancer I've heard that one can become depressed and I think that is something to look out for. The brightness of life we may have felt going through our ordeal dims over time, the dance fades, the steps forgotten. But this is okay and natural to forget although I doubt anyone forgets their cancer completely. Even in remission we know that next checkup may bring bad news. So we are slightly on the edge of our seat the rest of our lives. If we've learned anything we continue to look deeper into ourselves and our beloved's eyes, hug more often with a tighter embrace, linger with the sunset, help the helpless.

I have an incurable cancer. Furthermore the cause has yet to be discovered so there's nothing I can do to avoid it coming back. At times I feel like a sitting duck. I suppose I will carry on as I did before but do it with Love Trust Gratitude and Healing for as long as I can. I hope if you find yourself in a similar situation you can as well.

I mentioned earlier that after I decided that I chose my parents a balance was restored including my memories growing up with them. Good memories I had forgotten came to the fore and I'm grateful to have them. I would like to end with one of them:

I was eight when my dad bought an old homestead in northern Minnesota. On it was a dilapidated barn, a workshop, a shed, an outhouse and a little two bedroom house that was in decent shape but the roof leaked. Among many other skills my dad was an excellent carpenter. Because he worked during the day we put in a few all nighters, as he was eager to get the house livable and the family moved in. I was his sleepy little helper fetching nails and shingles and holding the end of the measuring tape. When I wasn't helping him I would slip into an old sleeping bag he tacked to the roof, so if I fell asleep I wouldn't roll off the pitched roof. I would lie in the sleeping bag gazing up at the stars, the Big Dipper, the glorious Milky Way, an occasional shooting star streaking across the sky, moths banging against the flood lights, bats zipping past, circling, zipping past again, swooping on the insects attracted by the lights. I would lose myself in the hypnotic sound of crickets in the grass below or the frogs from the wetlands croaking anonymously, before being interrupted by my dad checking in on me, "You okay over there?" Or calling me back to work, "Hey, get up and give me a hand over here will ya."

Over the period of a few weeks the experience ignited in me a deep love and appreciation for nature and the mystery of the stars. After we moved in I was out every night after dark chasing fireflies, searching for salamanders in the wet grass with a flashlight or spotlighting the trees trying in vain to locate an owl hooting in the dark woods, jumping at the sound of a stick snapping under the foot or paw of something scary that sent me scrambling back to the steps of the backdoor, staring into the dark beyond the yard light, listening intently for another sign from the unknown beast lurking out there. I remember one night a bear came into the yard and chased our dog around the house. This is likely an event where the bear would have been shot but my dad rushed out to bring the dog inside and let the bear wander away on its own. For all his faults I never saw my dad kill anything other than a weasel that was killing the chickens and even then he felt bad about it. There are catastrophes that engulf people and they cannot escape the effects even after decades or an entire lifetime. Perhaps my dad had suffered such a devastating childhood he couldn't heal enough to pass it on to me directly but did so indirectly through actions he took in his life.

These experiences from childhood prepared me for an ever uncertain future that laid ahead and I relied on them many times over the years especially when it came to facing my cancer with Love Trust Gratitude and Healing.

Epilogue

Cancer was a shocking turn of events that none of us were ready for. The initial impact blocked out the sun and I'll bet it is much the same for everyone who is thrust into this position. This is something for which we cannot prepare. Nothing about it was easy. It was a profound physical, emotional and spiritual confrontation. Yet overall it had a lightness to it. I think it is the aliveness I felt after I found myself on the floor confronting cancer. I said it before, now I'll say it one last time, cancer woke me up. The pain was temporary. The depth has remained.

Physically I've changed significantly. My guess is I've recovered around eighty percent of my former ability to walk. I'm clumsier than I was before. I have to give more attention to walking than I used to. Considering where I was at the start of this journey I'm okay with that. And there's more time for improvement though progress has slowed. I still have the band of numbness around my midsection and it's probably the thing that bothers me most, as it is often uncomfortable. It's a constant reminder of where I've been if I ever have an inkling to forget. There's still some numbness in my legs and feet. I don't have that former spring in my step. I'm told these may be permanent. I'm still not used to my curly hair. Sometimes when I absentmindedly touch my head I mistake a curl for a spider or something and panic trying to brush it off only to realize it's just a curl. I laugh out loud every time this happens. Life is wonderful.

Cancer was an opportunity to make peace with my death before my death and hopefully well before my death. Making peace with my death has been the path to living more fully. Cancer was also an opportunity to heal emotionally and spiritually beyond my pre-cancer self. The amount of that healing was determined by the quality of my response. I no longer fear my death.

I still meditate on Love Trust and Gratitude every day because I know it brings me Healing. I say this nine months out from my bone marrow transplant, so I'm not here to tell you I will survive this ordeal I'm going through because the jury is still out. It's the emotional and spiritual healing that I'm speaking of. As a culture we have become masters of the physical dimension but we lack utterly when it comes to the emotional and spiritual dimensions. Without them we are rampaging the planet in pursuit of our physical comforts and conveniences. Our satisfaction with objects is temporary so we go on to pursue other objects repeating until death. It is not uncommon for a man to reach the end of his life knowing more about his collection of cars than his wife's heart or his children's dreams. This is a tragedy.

Material gain beyond a modest amount is unfulfilling yet the every day message we receive is that more is better. It's difficult to change unless it comes in the form of a confrontation because the busy day-to-day and our natural aversion to change lulls us to sleep. We judge our lives and others on external things like houses, cars, positions, vacations, accomplishments, appearances. Then something like cancer comes along and suddenly our mortality is looming. If there are too few emotional and spiritual provisions laid away our suffering can be great. We suffer over our suffering. With little to rely on in terms of perspective we frame the experience as a battle and ourselves as warriors. If the war turns and the battle is lost we become victims. This goes to the heart of this book and my experience with cancer. By choosing dance over war and meditating on

Love Trust Gratitude Healing my experience with cancer was different from what it would have been had I chosen to deny it was happening, raged against it, or suffered over my suffering. We are the sum of our actions. As a country we spend nearly a trillion dollars a year on our military. We declare war on everything and everybody we don't like or understand. We are saturated in the language of war. We don't even notice how insane and futile something like a 'war on terror' is. Because war is terror what we're actually engaged in is a terror on terror. Making a bigger mess of a mess is a low quality response. The bottom line is, it isn't working for us. It is time for new metaphors for our encounters with cancer, the planet, each other.

I believe the idea of progress to a perfect world in the future is a mistake because it is the challenges and imperfections in life that give it meaning. Even when it comes to curing cancer that would be the case. I'm thinking of Dr. Appelbaum who has spent a lifetime studying blood cancers. From one point of view it can be said that it is his confrontation with cancer through research and investigation that has given his life meaning. Indeed it is likely the case for most of the folks working on these dreadful diseases. What would happen if all of them were suddenly cured? It would certainly be good news. However, something else would surely take its place. If not, a substantial purpose of life would vanish. We think what we want in life is a perfect hassle-free existence where everything falls into place. The truth is it would bore us to tears. What we really want from life is adventure. Of course we think we prefer a great adventure of certainty where everything is sure to end okay but this isn't true because it's the uncertainty and risk that makes every adventure worth undergoing. In other words if we knew the end of an adventure we wouldn't bother to pursue it in the first place. So, what we really want in life, the adventure and the uncertainty of it, is exactly what we get.

Exercises Worth Repeating

I was in the emergency room when I realized that Love, Trust, Gratitude, Healing were not just four nice words strung together but an equation or recipe. Put this way, Love + Trust + Gratitude = Healing. Or as a recipe: Love, Trust, and Gratitude are the ingredients and Healing is the result. For folks with a more traditional religious outlook Faith may be substituted for Trust: Love Faith Gratitude Healing.

My primary goal in dealing with the day to day struggle involved with cancer treatments was remaining calm and relaxed. My intuition was that this was the best state of being for helping the medicines do their job most effectively. Remaining calm and relaxed was especially difficult for treatments that were on the horizon where it was easy to get ahead of myself and start worrying about how they would affect my body and whether they were going to help or not. I found that meditating on Love Trust Gratitude and Healing really helped. They are effective simply because they take you out of your fear-laden speculative mind and shift you to the present as you think about the people, places and things in your life that you love, have gratitude for… If you're going through a crisis of your own and you're stuck in your speculative mind worrying about the future give them a try. I wish you great luck and great health.

Also, Jen and I added a visual element, writing Love Trust Gratitude Healing on pieces of poster board with color markers, adding a few creative touches and hanging them on the wall in our bedroom.

Exercise No. 1 for LTGH

The first exercise is to breathe deeply and repeat Love, Trust, Gratitude, Healing, slowly like a mantra. I found this simple exercise to be effective at redirecting my thoughts whenever my mind drifted into fearful speculation about the future.

Exercise No. 2 for LTGH

Pause on each word and list everyone you love, everything and everyone you trust, who and what you're grateful for: the people, the times, the places. The gratitude you feel for life and everyone who shares it with you. List the healing you desire and everyone you know who may be in need of healing. You can include everyone like I do because I really believe it's true for everyone whether it's emotional, spiritual or physical. Love Trust Gratitude Healing was an antidote for all the uncertainty, fear and speculation that accompanied my cancer diagnosis and the treatments that followed.

Here is a shorthand of my meditation:

Love: I love myself, I love my family (name them), I love my friends (name them), I love my community, I love everyone.

Trust: I trust myself to know what's right for me, I trust my family to help, I trust my medical team, I trust their research, their expertise.

Gratitude: I'm grateful for my life, the lives of my family, for all the people in my life, for my medical team, for the hard work and brilliant minds I will never meet who found a way to extend my life. I'm grateful for more life.

Healing: I'm in need of healing. My family is in need of healing, my community is in need of healing, everyone is in need of some form healing. The planet is in need of healing.

Exercise No. 3 for LTGH

This exercise takes the previous one and goes deeper meditating on what you Love about each person, place or thing on your list including yourself. Do the same with Trust, Gratitude and Healing.

Note: I found that writing down my answers for the second and third exercises helped when I was chemo-dosed and not thinking clearly. Then I could just read what I had already written.

Exercise No. 3 for LTGH

Acknowledgements

I am grateful for all the folks I crossed paths with at Seattle Cancer Care Alliance (SCCA) and the University of Washington Medical Center (UWMC) on the journey through my cancer diagnosis and subsequent treatments. As a patient they've done right by me every step of the way. I found everyone I encountered to be professional, informative and caring. They deserve the lion's share of credit for helping me heal physically. I would especially like to thank my oncologist Dr. Cowan and his team at SCCA. Also, the Aqua team who oversaw my bone marrow transplant. I couldn't have asked for a better group of professionals. They are engaged in meaningful work at it shows. I would also like to acknowledge all patients who have gone through this ordeal before me and from whose experience knowledge was gained and treatments were improved.

There is no way I could have gotten through this without the love and support of my family. My wife Jen was incredible carrying the load and in the early going literally carrying me. Our daughter Ocean, her husband Troy, and our son Bluewolf were incredibly strong and resilient. Our neighbors Sally and Dan Benson went above and beyond supporting us through my illness. I would like to thank everyone who read my manuscript and gave great feedback and encouragement. A big thank you to Ross Baarslag-Benson for his careful reading of my manuscript and valuable editing suggestions.

LOVE TRUST GRATITUDE HEALING

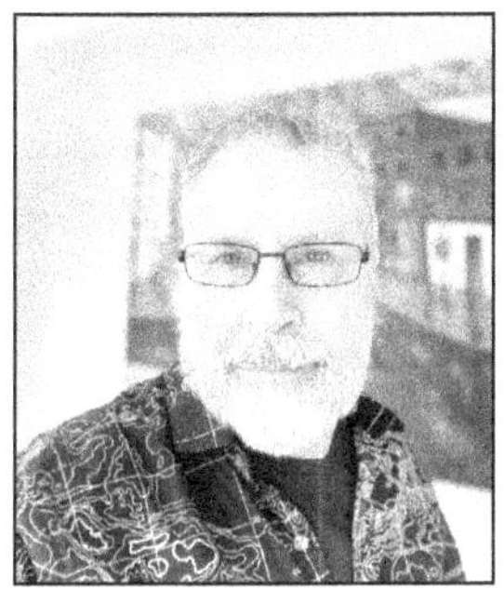

Michael McDaeth is a musician and writer living in Seattle. He is the author of two novels *Roads and Parking Lots* and *Under Protest*. He has written and recorded hundreds of songs over the years as a solo artist, and with his band Weeds, garnering an international following. Michael has a few dozen short films to his credit ranging from animation, stop-motion, found footage to mixed-media. As a freelance writer Michael has published short stories, poetry, and creative essays.

www.lovetrustgratitudehealing.com
www.mcdaeth.com

* 9 7 9 8 6 8 9 3 1 6 0 3 1 *